JOHN KILLICK was a teacher f
been a writer all his life. He h
his own poetry and books or
began working with people with dementia in 1992,
and has held a number of posts with nursing homes,
hospitals, libraries and arts centres. With Kate Allan,
John created and moderates the website www.dementia-
positive.co.uk. He has edited six books of poems by
people with dementia, and co-authored books on
communication and on creativity. He has written many
articles and book chapters, and given many workshops
in the UK and abroad. He has also made a number of
appearances on radio and TV.

THE
STORY OF DEMENTIA

JOHN KILLICK

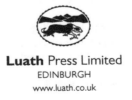

Luath Press Limited
EDINBURGH
www.luath.co.uk

First published 2017

ISBN: 978-1-912147-05-2

The paper used in this book is recyclable. It is made from
low chlorine pulps produced in a low energy, low emission
manner from renewable forests.

Printed and bound by
Bell & Bain Ltd., Glasgow

Typeset in 10.5 point Sabon and Gill
by 3btype.com

CONTENTS

For Kerry and Richard of the
Australian Journal of Dementia Care
for all their support.

COLLAGE OF EXPRESSIONS TO BE MET WITH IN THE
MEDIA

Help Beat Dementia

The Rising Tide

A LIVING DEATH

The Burden of Alzheimer's

A Silent Tsunami

An Epidemic of Mental Impairment

A Challenge for Champions

THE QUIET CRISIS

A Spreading Contagion

Leading the Fight Against Dementia

A TIME-BOMB

FULL HUMANITY

Subject Rather Than Object

Hearing the Voice

Nothing About Us Without Us

**Not Person with DEMENTIA
but PERSON with Dementia**

Living Positively

Active Listening

The Cry of Solidarity
and the Demand for Citizenship

Back-up Brains

Design For Disability

I Feel and Relate Therefore I Am

We have the Dementia We Deserve

John Killick came to the field of dementia care quite late in his life and brought mature eyes to bear on the experiences of people with dementia and the approaches to their care. His skills as an observer, communicator and poet were well honed and were put at the service of an intensely empathic nature. The result has been a series of books of poetry that have enabled the reader to feel the joys and fears of many, very real, people who have dementia. These books clearly show that John is well equipped to see beyond the platitudes often used to describe the world of the person with dementia, a world that is affected by the efforts of researchers, practitioners and clinicians as they strive to find ways to be of help.

In *The Story of Dementia* John has turned his attention to these experts and applied his empathic understanding of the experiences of people with dementia to identify those that have made a genuine contribution to their care and wellbeing. He has dug into their writings to find the gems of their understanding and shows them to us with a clarity that is very hard to achieve in such brief chapters. General readers who have never read an article or a text book on dementia will find their interest piqued as John brings out the motivations behind each author's writings and shows how they have made a particular contribution to the field. John knows more than most that we have a long way to go before we can claim to understand either the process of dementia or the experience of people with dementia. However, this lively book will open doors to what we do know, providing immediately available insights to the casual reader and references to the sources for those who wish to dig deeper.

I believe that inclusion in this book should be taken as a great honour. John is very capable of separating the wheat from the chaff.

Professor Richard Fleming
Executive Director
Dementia Training Australia
University of Wollongong
Australia

This book tells a story without an ending. Some may think it is rather premature to tell it at all since we may well still be near the beginning. But in my view it needs telling, even in a truncated form, since it is a complicated picture and some way needs to be found to identify a kind of a pattern in it.

Why should I be the person to attempt it? Well, because I am a writer, not a researcher, or a professional, or a family carer, or a person with dementia, and to that extent can stand outside it. On the other hand, in this instance I am not just a professional writer who can pick up a subject, write about it, then put it down again and move on to the next topic. When this book appears I shall have been working in the dementia field for a full quarter of a century, predominantly directly with people with dementia in care homes, day centres, hospitals and their own homes. I have concentrated on the twin aspects of communication and creativity and already published extensively on these. I have met ten of the twelve subjects of these chapters, and many more who might have been included. I have attended conferences and seminars and read widely on the subject. I have formed opinions and believe I have attained a perspective.

Of course, there are people working in dementia who will not share that perspective. This is inevitable in an area where so little is known, and so many are travelling hopefully without any reassuring sense of arrival. The academic world is split, with individuals and groups often adhering to diametrically opposed theories and practices. They are unlikely to be reconciled until understanding reaches a more secure level, and the truth when it comes will almost certainly partake of both viewpoints.

The plan I have adopted is a straightforward one. I have chosen 12 individuals to represent the field of enquiry, and hope that in general terms they represent different areas of expertise, but I do not regard this as pigeon-holing; the individuals come first, and their specialisms second. I readily recognise the choice is a personal one, and others might have selected different contributors to the scene, maybe with a wider international scope. I write from within my own limitations in this regard.

The format, then, is simple, the arguments less so. I have tried to write as comprehensibly as possible. Some subjects are too convoluted to explain in words of one syllable, let alone two. I have kept the chapters short. Anyone wanting to follow up a person's take on any particular aspect should read the books, chapters and papers listed. I have put the references at the end of the book to keep the main text uncluttered.

The one exception to the short chapters rule is Number Five. This is the one in which people with the condition hold sway. Listening to the voices of those experiencing dementia occupies a crucial position in learning about the subject, and has been much neglected by self-styled 'experts', so I make no apology for allocating them a little more space than anyone else.

The overall message of the book is hopeful. In this, I feel, it offers a contrast to much of what the media presents us with: a kind of fairground ride of lows and highs. The lows are the negativity of fear and disaster promulgated by headlines emphasising numbers of people being diagnosed; 'tsunamis of dementia' are conjured up which threaten to sink our societies beneath the waves. The highs are equally exaggerated: taking a particular pill or following a diet or regime of exercise are heralded in tall front-page headlines as saving us from extinction. My claims are modest, a cautiously optimistic picture of the future is painted by the individuals I have chosen to feature. So the story of dementia as I present it in these pages is the alternative narrative which has been occupying the shadowlands of the subject, and which is much in need of bringing into the light.

I have benefited from the advice of some of the subjects of this book, who have commented on my writings, but must stress that fundamentally the responsibility for the text, with all its shortcomings, is mine alone.

John Killick

Of all the pages in this book, this is the most difficult to write, because no-one can agree on a precise form of words.

Professor Julian Hughes (see Chapter Eight) favours 'acquired diffuse neurological dysfunction', whereas the American Psychiatric Association in the new-minted 5th edition of their 'Diagnostic and Statistical Manual of Mental Disorders' has plumped for 'a neuro-cognitive disorder'.

Closer to home, the National Health Service goes for 'a syndrome (a group of related symptoms) associated with an ongoing decline of the brain' and the Alzheimer's Association prefers 'a general term for a decline in mental ability severe enough to interfere with daily life'.

Personally, I would reject all these negative and wholly medicalised viewpoints in favour of something which emphasised multiple causes and consequences, and which gave equal weight to the biological on the one hand, and the psychological and social, aspects on the other.

No doubt infuriated by the fear and stigma aroused by the word, Professor Carol Brayne of Oxford University would abolish it altogether and just talk about 'brain ageing'!

Over one million people in the UK are expected to be diagnosed with dementia by 2025, a number expected to double by 2051

62% of those diagnosed with dementia are affected by Alzheimer's disease, making it the most common diagnosis

35.6 million people worldwide are affected by dementia

Three quarters of people with dementia worldwide have not received a diagnosis – per one study, in India the undiagnosed could total 90%

25,000 people from BAME backgrounds in the UK are affected

1 in every 14 of the population aged 65 and over in the UK is affected by dementia

1 in 3 people in the UK will care for a person with dementia in their lifetime

£11 billion is saved by the labour of unpaid carers in the UK every year

66,000 people have cut their working hours to care for someone with dementia, and 50,000 have left work altogether

£4.5 billion worth of costs of dementia in the UK is picked up by the NHS

£50 million is going to be spent on the UK's first dedicated Dementia Research Institute

Five times fewer researchers choose to work on dementia than on cancer

72% of those with dementia live with another condition or disability, most commonly arthritis, hearing problems, heart disease or a physical disability

25% of hospital beds are estimated to be occupied by those with dementia

40% of people with dementia report feeling lonely

34% do not feel part of their community

One third of people with dementia live in a care home

Over one million Dementia Friends have been recruited since Public Health England and Alzheimer's Society launched the campaign in 2014

13,583 people with dementia were forecasted to take part in dementia research in 2013/14, improving on 2012/13 by almost 1%

Every three minutes someone in the UK develops dementia

55% of people living with dementia are in the mild stages

56% of people put off seeking a diagnosis for a year or more

62% of people feel that a diagnosis of dementia means that their life is over.

CHAPTER ONE

The Identifier

Alois Alzheimer

For the beginning of the story I am going back to 1906. That is not to say that dementia, in one form or another, did not exist before that date, but that was the year the condition we now refer to as Alzheimer's was first identified.

It is called Alzheimer's because that was the name of the person who first made the discovery – Alois Alzheimer. The person to whom he first attached the title was Frau Auguste D. It came about like this: Alois was a doctor who, in 1888, obtained a post as Assistant Medical Officer at the Municipal Mental Hospital in Frankfurt, Germany. In 1901 Frau D was admitted to the hospital with complex psychological symptoms. Alois became deeply interested in her case, and when he left the hospital in 1903 to take up positions in Heidelberg and Munich he entered into an agreement with the asylum that, upon her death, Frau D's brain would be sent to him for analysis.

Frau D died in 1906 (she was only 55) and thus it was that Alois embarked upon a piece of research that proved to be of historical significance. At that time, the all-embracing category for older people with mental health problems was 'senile dementia', but Alois claimed to have discovered a variant of this, characterised by plaques and tangles (these are prime suspects in cell death and tissue loss in the brain, which Alois studied on slides under a microscope). Later that year he delivered a three-page paper in the form of a case study to the South-West German Association of Psychiatrists identifying a distinctive pathology on the basis of this one example. Thus the disease 'belonging to Alzheimer' was born.

All that's true, but we can't underestimate the importance of another academic, Ernst Kraepelin, who held professorships at the Universities of Heidelberg and Munich during Alois' time at both institutions, and to whom Alois was indebted for his mentorship.

During that decade there were other researchers looking at dementia who could easily have come to the fore. Kraepelin, however, chose to promote Alois' work in the textbook he published. It was already a well-thumbed tome, and it was in the 1910 edition (the eighth!) that he created this subdivision of 'senile dementia'. The professor, we may surmise, was engaged in an exercise of academic one-upmanship, to keep his university ahead of its rivals, and Alois' discovery was grist to his mill. 'Alzheimer's Disease' was now officially on the map.

Only it wasn't really, as we shall see. Alois was a modest sort of man, not given to self-promotion, and not interested in fame. He wasn't interested in fortune either as he had a private income. Our knowledge of his personality is scant, but here is a description which gives us some insight:

> From 1903 to 1912, his years in Munich, Alzheimer
> became a well-loved figure to students from all over
> the world. He would spend hours with each one,
> explaining things as they shared a microscope, always
> with a cigar that would be put down as he
> commenced his explanations, and it is said that at the

end of the day there would always be a cigar stump at
every student's bench by the microscope.[1]

One might have imagined that the trajectory of knowledge about dementia and the universal use of the term
'Alzheimer's' would have proceeded steadily from 1910,
but this was far from the case. There was little awareness that anything significant had occurred, and perhaps
the shock of two world wars had something to do
with the lack of follow-up. The term might never have
come into general circulation if the steady increase in
life expectancy had not had repercussions on mental
health. Yet even in 1970, Brendan Maher in his book
Principles of Psychopathology[2] was to state 'Alzheimer's
Disease is statistically infrequent and of little interest to
students of psychopathology'. By 1983 it was impossible to ignore the effects of demographic change, so
in Australia, Scott Henderson[3] could publish an article
entitled *The Coming Epidemic of Dementia*, whilst in
1989 in Britain Robert Woods[4] was authoring a book
Alzheimer's Disease: Coping with a Living Death. Today
it is impossible to escape the name of the man who
bears the condition's name: it is on everyone's lips.
Many have little idea of its origin or meaning, but it
has the capacity to instil dread.

This escalation probably first occurred in America.
There the medicalisation of old age really took hold.
The DSM (Diagnostic and Statistical Manual of Mental
Disorders) emanating from the American Psychiatric
Association enshrined the condition as holy writ in 1980,
and it was seized upon by Alzheimer's Associations in

various countries and internationally, in conjunction with drugs companies, as a means of raising funds.

But we still need to pause and consider. How can it be that all this paraphernalia of papers, books, conferences, broadcasts and organisations has stemmed from the observations of one doctor of one patient? It is something that certainly could not occur in the 21st century. Our research methods are not only much more sophisticated, but our scepticism is much more highly developed. Aggregation is the name of the game: we employ teams of specialists with their batteries of tests before even the most tentative hypothesis is advanced. The only conclusion that could possibly be reached is that Alois was onto something.

And of course he was. We still employ similar tests to those he carried out with similar results leading to similar conclusions. But there the problems begin to arise. In considering how Frau D presented, did Alois explore all the options? Or did he overlook possibilities which might have led to different conclusions?

Here is part of the description offered by Alois in his original account:

> Following institutionalisation she appeared totally bewildered. She was disoriented as to time and place and occasionally stated that she did not understand events around her. She treated her physician as a guest, excused herself and said she was not finished with her work. Following this she would scream aloud that he was trying to stab her with a knife, or indignantly turn him away, fearing that he would violate her. She was

intermittently delirious, dragging her bedding about, called for her husband and daughter, and appeared to be having auditory hallucinations. She would scream for hours in a monstrous voice.[5]

At the time when Alois was coming to the conclusion that Frau D had a specific form of dementia, Sigmund Freud was advocating a psychoanalytic approach (his *Studies in Hysteria* had been published in 1895[6]) We can only speculate how he would have proceeded faced with her behaviour. There is no evidence that Alois inquired into Frau D's life history. Had she been sexually abused? When he came to do his post-mortem work did he take into account her nearly five-year incarceration? Was she schizophrenic? Was she subject to bouts of depression? Were there any other medical conditions which might have contributed to her predicament? The fact that she was younger than those people normally classified as having 'senile dementia' might have alerted him to the possibility that different factors entirely may have been operative in her decline.

In their book *Understanding Dementia: The Man with the Worried Eyes* Rick Cheston and Mike Bender[7] challenge in a number of ways the accepted view of the diagnosis made by Alois, and I am indebted to them for the list in the previous paragraph. Their conclusion is:

> We have discussed possible alternative explanations of Frau Auguste D's condition. We hope we have also shown how the 'great man/inevitability of scientific progress' frame does not fit well with the actual history of Alzheimer's disease.

Here Cheston and Bender are calling into question the whole reputation of Alois as a pioneer of dementia research. It is incontrovertible, though, that his work, for good or ill, has had a massive influence on all that has occurred in the field up to the present-day. We need to examine this legacy further.

Because Alois took an entirely biomedical view of the individual he was studying, and entirely neglected what we may call the psychosocial aspects (which is something for which he can be held responsible), and because the clinical establishment seized upon the former and created a massive superstructure of ideas and procedures upon its flimsy foundation over the past half-century (for which he cannot be held responsible), it has become necessary to establish a counter-culture to restore the balance. Most of the rest of the history of dementia theory and practice reflects this movement. It also has to be admitted that, following Alois' example of analysis, with its consequent concentration on seeking a cure largely through developing drug treatments, has not exactly led to conspicuous success.

The psychologist Tom Kitwood states:

> The whole conceptual framework of biomedical research into dementia ... is far from adequate to the problem field ... It is necessary to have a paradigm in order to focus attention on particular problems. This paradigm, however, does not provide a sound basis for the general explanation of dementia – Alzheimer's or any other type. It is logically flawed, and it does not easily accommodate the full range of evidence. p8

Whilst acknowledging Alois' significance, Kitwood goes on to list his provisos, before then proceeding to unfold his alternative scenarios. This will be the subject of the next chapter.

CHAPTER TWO

The Visionary

Tom Kitwood

In Chapter One I prepared the way for this one by claiming that Tom Kitwood was the man who brought new insights to the story of dementia and pointed the way forward for psychosocial research and practice.

Tom was a Senior Lecturer in counselling, psychotherapy and depth psychology at the University of Bradford, UK, before he became interested in dementia. His first book published in 1970 was called *What is Human*[1] and it was his concentration upon answering that question which informed his contribution to the dementia field. He was a challenging writer and a charismatic lecturer, but above all he immersed himself in practical communication with individuals with the condition, and observation of how family and professional carers coped with day-to-day domestic and institutional life respectively.

Out of this came his one substantial book on the subject *Dementia Reconsidered: the person comes first.*[2] In 1998 he was appointed Alois Alzheimer Professor of Psychogerontology at the University, but he was dead within the year. The academic post's title had a somewhat ironic twist, since he had already done much to put Alois in his place, distinctly lower in the pecking order than the one he had occupied before.

Dementia Reconsidered is an extraordinary achievement, a time bomb lobbed into the middle of the dementia establishment. The condition could never be seen in the same way again. Yet it is a short book, barely 150 pages, packed with explosive ideas.

Tom first of all mounts a demolition of dependence on the medical model. He attacks what he terms 'the standard paradigm' – the idea that dementia has entirely physical origins, and all its mental and emotional effects are directly the result of brain deterioration. He also attempts to undermine the concept of causation as a straight line of cause and effect, postulating instead a nexus of interacting factors.

And he draws attention to the different pace at which the condition develops in different individuals, and how there may be explanations for this which involve personal and social experiences which the biomedical approach takes no account of. He characterises the model as a mechanical structure ignoring the real lives of people, and offering no guidance as to how we should respond to them as human beings.

This critique of determinism, in his view, clears the way for a multifaceted approach to dementia, in which we can offer practical advice rather than technical explanation, hope rather than despair. He unfolds a whole range of aspects to be considered:

> culture, locality, social class, education, financial resources, the availability or absence of support and services. Also, at the interpersonal or social-psychological level, much depends on how far a person with dementia is enabled to retain intact relationships, to use his or her abilities, to experience variety and enjoyment. p37/8

Suddenly, in these words, he blows wide a door to dementia which had remained firmly closed since Alois made his discovery. It is almost impossible to estimate the significance of this achievement, or the effect it would have on later theory and practice.

But Tom does not stop with pronouncements; he is determined to show how these concepts can provide tools for humanising care. But first of all he confronts another slap in the face of those living with dementia: the awful unpreparedness of society for dealing with the challenges and opportunities it presents. He traces the unenlightened attitudes of Europe through the centuries to those with serious mental health issues, which has left countries without positive strategies or empathetic attitudes when dementia came to be identified. He leaves us in no doubt that a sea-change in moral responsibility is called for.

He proceeds to spell out what this means at the microcosmic level. He speaks of a 'malignant social psychology' which permeates our approach to people with the condition, whether in the home or the institution, and identifies no fewer than 17 categories of offences committed; these include disempowerment, stigmatisation, infantilisation, outpacing, ignoring and mockery. Overall looms the general characteristic of neglect, the deprivation of people with dementia of basic human contact, rendering them almost in the category of pariahs.

In order to demonstrate to those without dementia the prevalence of these patterns of behaviour, Tom devised an operational method of observation and evaluation termed 'Dementia Care Mapping'. This involves using a categorisation system to record examples of positive and negative behaviour of individuals with dementia in a care setting. It can then be used to classify a unit as helpful or destructive in atmosphere and practice, and also to the staff of where they are succeeding and going wrong in relation to those in their care.

Tom unfolds the concept of 'person-centred care' and makes much use of the term 'personhood', which he defines as:

> a standing or status that is bestowed upon one human being by others, in the context of relationship and social being. It implies recognition, respect and trust. Both the according of personhood and the failure to do so, have consequences which are empirically testable. p8

In another passage he claims:

> The time has come to recognise men and women who have dementia in their full humanity. Our frame of reference should no longer be person-with-DEMENTIA but PERSON-with-dementia. p7

In his outline of possible ways forward Tom encompasses many developments which have since occurred to a greater or lesser degree. He was remarkably prescient: he foresaw innovations in reminiscence, the arts, stimulation of the senses, and individual counselling and group therapy, for example. He illustrates his projections with a number of concrete or invented examples of positive caring practices. He summarises his reasons for optimism in the words:

> ... the general inference to be drawn from research to
> date is how much has been achieved through
> interventions that are only relatively modest; if
> improvements were consistent and throughout the
> entire context of dementia, we might reasonably
> expect to see much more than this. We are very far
> from having reached the limits that are genuinely set
> by the structural state of the brain. p64

He even suggests 'rementing' – the idea that by a variety of therapeutic provision the development of a dementia can not only be halted but actually reversed.

Another innovative approach which Tom proposes, and which has had far-reaching effects, is that instead of generalising about people with dementia and how they might feel about their condition and the care offered to them, it might be possible to consult them and act upon their views. In 1997 this was still quite a revolutionary suggestion! Now, though in some quarters it still has an air of novelty, generally it is accepted that this is a workable idea. And with some organisations run by people with the condition themselves it has resulted in the mantra 'Nothing for us without us'.

Tom first of all asserts that everyone is a unique individual and should be respected as such. He enumerates some of the ways in which they may be encountered. There is first of all their written accounts, as distinct from those composed by carers; at that time there were barely a handful of these – now we can pick and choose amongst a dozen or two. Then he proposes interviews and groupwork; this too was in its infancy, and now is attempted widely. Next there is close listening in informal situations, and he acknowledges that this may involve interpretation of symbolic language. Movement and gesture form another viable approach. Questioning people who have experienced similar but parallel medical or psychological conditions is a further mode of inquiry. Assisting people to compose poetry is a sixth strategy to be addressed and can result in memorable insights. Finally Tom advocates role-play as a means of simulating the condition; many who attended his presentations can attest to the power of his own practice of this approach. In all these ways he shone a searchlight on communication as a key element of care.

Another area Tom examines in the book is an answer to the question: 'What do people with dementia need?' He comes up with the following: comfort, attachment, inclusion, occupation and identity. He groups them together under the central concept of love. He is challenging us here with the fundamentals of his humanistic psychology.

Tom devotes forty pages of his short book to proposals for improving care. There is a chapter in which he analyses the components of care. This includes a consideration of the various types of interaction. In a key passage he finds a potent metaphor for what is required:

> We might imagine a natural forest of conifers, interspersed with patches of alpine meadow in which

a hundred species are to be found in a few square yards. Poor care, in contrast, is dead and regimented; there are long periods of neglect, and small episodes of malignant social psychology fill a few of the spaces. We might think of a conifer plantation cultivated purely for the purposes of agribusiness, where the trees are in rows and almost nothing grows between them; there is virtually no sign of the grace and beauty of a natural system, and the atmosphere is dark and depressing. p93

In his chapter on institutions he castigates those content with a soulless environment, and lauds those which bring 'positive person-work' to the fore, whilst acknowledging the demands this places on the attentiveness of the caregivers. He pays attention to the qualities necessary for this kind of demanding work, and stresses the importance of caring for the staff as well as the residents.

He ends his book with a characterisation of the 'Old and New Cultures of Care', and an acknowledgement of the powerful forces resisting change, which training and example urgently need to address.

It is inevitable that in the years since the publication of Tom's book it in its turn should have been subjected to various critiques, even though the fundamental orientation of his ideas has been largely accepted. There is room for mention of four of these here. One is the fundamentally psychological tenor of his approach. It is claimed that he neglects the wider societal and economic movements which provide the context in which dementia flourishes and care is held back. Then his concept of personhood has been challenged as too limited in its scope, lacking awareness of power issues in relation to individuals or groups which may result in the withdrawal of recognition. Thirdly, his idea of relationships has seemed to some to lack coherence, insufficiently stressing the importance of quality in his descriptions. Lastly, his understanding of real-life care settings has been questioned, with too great a reliance on schematic or formulaic models. The most thoroughgoing examination of Kitwood's writings yet to appear (including the consideration of papers which expand on ideas promulgated in the book) is that by Clive Baldwin and Andrea Capstick.[3]

Notwithstanding the numerous provisos which have piled up in the two decades since the publication of *Dementia Reconsidered*, it remains the seminal text for those involved in the fight-back to establish a truly psychosocial approach, and all the subjects of the succeeding chapters remain deeply in his debt.

CHAPTER THREE

The Polymath

Mary Marshall

After Alois Alzheimer and Tom Kitwood, all the other individuals in this personalised history series are alive and mostly still active in the field. This itself is a sign of how far we have come in disseminating the ideas which Tom was the first to articulate. Of them all Mary Marshall has had by far the widest scope and influence over a whole range of topics and approaches. She is truly the polymath of the psychosocial movement. Her contributions encompass theory, research and practice, and she has had a significant impact on both public and private spheres.

Mary began as a social worker, but on the way gained experience as a university lecturer. It was a visit to Australia in 1982, when she was on a sabbatical and worked there in a hospital for people with dementia, that her interest in the subject was aroused. She was blown away by evidence of a psychosocial model in action (small households in normal housing, specially designed units and community based day care) – such a contrast to the almost wholly medically-based care in Britain at that time. She returned inspired, and left her Liverpool University post to head up Age Concern Scotland, which chose dementia as its theme in 1986. This led to the formation of Scottish Action on Dementia, a highly successful lobbying group. In 1997 Mary wrote:

> Until ten or so years ago it [dementia care] was characterised by profound therapeutic nihilism. The combination of characteristics: old age, challenging behaviour, incompetence, loss of insight, low status,

increasing numbers and poor success in pharmacological research cast a deep shadow.[1]

She indicated some of the positives in the current scene as hearing the effective voice of carers, the beginnings of personal accounts from some people with the condition, and the burgeoning of professional literature, particularly that influenced by Kitwood's concepts. Scottish Action found that it was getting numerous requests for information and training and saw the need for a Dementia Services Development Centre. Every academic institution in Scotland was invited to bid for it, Edinburgh and Stirling were shortlisted, and Stirling won. Mary was persuaded to apply for the post of Director. The embedding in a university gave it academic clout, but as a service body it also needed to be at arm's length from the often stultifying conservatism of such an institution. A bipartite arrangement was favoured – a charity embedded in a university department. Thus, in 1989 the Dementia Services Development Centre at the University of Stirling was born. It was a novel solution, and an uncomfortable one at times, but on the whole served Mary well over the 16 years of her tenure as its manager and inspirer. It was funded partly by the Scottish Office and partly by grants from other public bodies and charities, often related to specific initiatives. When Mary retired in 2005 she left behind a vibrant, ground-breaking team with an international reputation for excellence. She had also established a model which came to be reproduced throughout the United Kingdom and abroad, especially in Australia where she had already forged close links. Her period of office had also been marked by connections and collaborations throughout Britain and abroad in a spirit of shared exploration.

At this point I have to declare an interest, for I worked under Mary for 12 of those years, and I can testify to the exciting collaborative atmosphere she engendered. Whilst always herself being in the forefront of identifying fresh areas for enquiry, and backing those which came from her staff, she was keenly interested in keeping abreast of those from other sources. Never a staff meeting passed without her asking the question 'What are the hot topics this month?' We would need to be aware of them and to formulate our plans for following them up.

Colleagues will testify that when presented with a new idea which seemed to have potential, Mary would both give active encouragement and autonomy to the initiator. As a writer employed by the Centre, itself an unusual appointment, I was offered the freedom to write and publish what I wanted in the Centre's name without censorship; this kind of trust, I believe, is unusual in managers, who are usually watching their backs for fear of reprisals.

Amongst the spectrum of topics which the Centre identified, investigated and published on were: acute hospitals, alcohol addiction, the arts, complementary therapies, deafness, learning disability, life-story work, sexuality and technology.

There were three areas of special achievement. In 1994 as a contribution to an Alzheimer's International Conference in Edinburgh Mary directed a half-day session on 'The Experience of Dementia', which brought together the various strands of relationships, therapeutic counselling and the arts in what was probably the first forum of its kind in the world, putting the voice of people with the condition in the forefront.

Politically Mary has always been active, and in 1999 the UK-wide Royal Commission on the Long-Term Care of Older People, of which she was a member, reported. Scotland set up a working group to consider the proposals, and Mary contributed to that too. As a result, Scotland is the only part of Britain to have adopted the recommendation of free personal care, which has left many family carers there in a better financial position than elsewhere.

In 2002 the Iris Murdoch Centre, to house the DSDC, was opened. This was the first purpose-built dementia-friendly building of its kind, which Mary had seen through from its first sketches.

Mary once said to me that, though it was probably unproveable, she believed that the development of a dementia owed more to environmental, social and personal factors than to any biological inheritance. All her work stemmed from this conviction.

Probably Mary's greatest passion in the dementia field is design. She sees failures in this area as one of the greatest factors leading to illbeing, and successes fundamental to living contentedly with the condition. However, she realises that the presentation of design principles is insufficient on its own to encourage best practice. There needs to be a wholesale acceptance of dementia as a disability for this to occur. In one of her first statements of this revolutionary idea she wrote:

> In terms of design it is really helpful to take a disability approach rather than a pathological one because disability is something for which design can compensate... Dementia as a disability is characterised by: impaired memory; impaired ability to learn; impaired ability to reason; high levels of stress[2]

She goes on to show how design can compensate for each of these disabilities in turn.

Mary perceived that there were good models of design in Australia, and it is no accident that her main book on this subject was written in collaboration with two Australians, Stephen Judd and Peter Phippen.[3]

In recent years she has turned her attention to exteriors of buildings – the gardens which surround or are attached to buildings. This has resulted in three major publications, one on her own,[4] one in collaboration with Annie Pollock,[5] and the last with Jane Gilliard.[6]

Ethical issues have also occupied Mary. The whole business of keeping people with dementia from harming themselves can easily go too far. In an article in 2005 she wrote:

> We talk too easily about risk assessment and risk management, but how often do we talk about the

risks of fundamentally diminishing a person's quality of life with our determination to avoid risk. I recall seeing a big, strong, younger man with dementia and a history of aggression, ironing happily in a psychiatric unit. Ironing is considered far too risky in most care homes.[7]

One of Mary's most significant edited books is *Perspectives on Rehabilitation and Dementia*, which also came out in 2005. A point she makes here, which shows her 'feet on the ground' stance, is the following:

One of the pressures in dementia care is to make it respectable, in the sense of making it mainstream, in the hope that people with dementia will cease to be marginalised. If we can label some of the dementia care 'rehabilitation', we stand some chance of mainstream healthcare both understanding and taking an interest in it.[8]

Mary has always embraced new technologies, both promoting them and subjecting them to critical scrutiny. She perceived early on their potential for helping people to maintain their independence and minimise the effects of their disability. Her *ASTRID: A guide to using technology within dementia care*[9] is required reading on this subject.

Although I have mentioned a number of books which Mary has edited rather than fully written herself, I have not adequately stressed her genius for collaboration, and the bringing together of a number of different authors on a subject. Three outstanding examples must be: *Food, Glorious Food: Perspectives on Food and Dementia*,[10] which gives equal weight to diet and the pleasures of eating. My own favourite is *Time for Dementia: A collection of writings on the meaning of time and dementia.*[11] As usual, the book's introduction, jointly written with the co-editor Jane Gilliard, does not eschew challenges:

> When we say we do not have time for 'person centred care', or 'spending time talking to people with dementia' or 'enabling them to do things for themselves even though it takes longer' – what are we really saying? Are we saying that spending time with a person with dementia has less value than a staff meeting for example, or tidying up? Time is the currency of dementia care; we spend it on what we value most.

Another book edited with Jane Gilliard is *Fresh Air on My Face: Transforming the quality of life for people with dementia through contact with the natural world.*[12] In a way this is the most obvious of all Mary's books, and at the same time the most revolutionary. It stems from indignation at the neglect of such an essential right. As the editors say:

> It never ceases to surprise us that this book is necessary because it is possible that people in many care homes never go outside... We are all part of nature and suffer if this connection is not reinforced all the time, or is even severed. We must have contact with nature for our physical, mental and physical health. People with dementia in care homes are fellow citizens and we all must ensure that they have the same opportunities as we have to relate to and be part of nature.

Of all Mary's edited books perhaps the one which most reflects the breadth of her concerns is one of the earliest – *The State of the Art in Dementia Care* in 1997 (1) In this she picked out some of the movers and shakers of the time, 50 in all, and gave each of them a limited number of words in which to put their case. This resulted in one of the most stimulating and readable contributions to the whole literature. It may be out of print, but it is certainly not out of relevance.

I hope the quotations from Mary's writings that I have chosen give some idea of her range and right-thinking clarity of expression. To sum up her legacy (still being added to), if Tom drew the outlines, Mary coloured in many of the pictures in the most pragmatic and practical terms – a true trailblazer.

CHAPTER FOUR

The Communicator

Steven Sabat

Tom Kitwood and Mary Marshall both saw communication as a cornerstone of care, and of those who have made a major contribution in this area I have chosen Steven Sabat as their representative. He is probably less well-known than other people featured in this series, and has written only one book, but that is a master work; his co-editing of another, and his various papers and chapters are ancillary to that achievement.

To those who haven't had the pleasure or privilege of meeting Steven, a glance at the acknowledgement pages in his book *The Experience of Alzheimer's Disease: Life Through a Tangled Veil*[1] will tell you what sort of a man he is. Never has an author acknowledged his sources of support more fulsomely. His students at Georgetown University in Washington, where he taught for 40 years and where he is now Emeritus Professor of Psychology, were fortunate indeed.

Before I begin outlining Steven's achievement I must register a small caveat. Throughout his book he freely employs the words 'sufferer' and 'afflicted' of people with dementia. For me these terms jar and tend to contradict his message, which is one of humanity and compassion.

In his preface Steven makes two crucial observations in view of what is to follow. The first identifies our responsibility towards a person with the condition, and the consequences of our dereliction of it:

> How we view the sufferer – as a human being whose sense of self, whose dignity, dispositions, pride, and whose ability to understand the meaning of situations

and to act meaningfully, remain intact to some degree on the one hand, or as a 'demented', defective, helpless and confused patient lacking a self, on the other – will affect the ways in which we treat that person, which in turn will affect how that person behaves.

The second is summed up in the words:

> This book represents a paradigm shift in that the afflicted person is seen as the <u>subject</u> of study rather than as an <u>object</u> of study.

Once that transition is accomplished it becomes possible to let 'the wealth of living reality'[2] in. It complicates the issue, of course, but this acts as a necessary corrective to mechanistic theorising.

From his experience as a psychologist, Steven noticed that his medical colleagues attributed errors in speech and understanding by people with dementia entirely to brain damage, whereas his instinct was to see them as misunderstandings of communication. As such they could be characteristics of both partners in an interaction. Since the medics could not provide a cure for the condition, he concluded that concentrating on the mistakes in reading language and situations by the parties might yield insights which could affect the quality of care. He determined to pursue this line of enquiry.

An example of what he meant was the phenomenon of what (borrowing the term from Social Psychology) he called 'Positioning'. This is best illustrated by an example:

> It was immediately following a talk I had given to caregivers that an intelligent and sensitive caregiver, and her spouse who was an AD sufferer, approached me with a few questions and comments. She began by thanking me for the lecture, and introduced herself. She then introduced her husband who was standing to her side and slightly behind her, by saying, 'This is my husband; he's the patient'. In this situation the spouse of the speaker was positioned immediately as an Alzheimer sufferer. p18

Positive and negative consequences of Positioning can result in an individual feeling:

> powerful or powerless, confident or apologetic, dominant or submissive, definitive or tentative, authorised or unauthorised[3]

These are distinctions which Steven draws in the first chapter of his book. Amongst the subjects covered by later chapters are: Language (the longest), Disability, Self-Esteem and Selfhood. These titles, however give no indication of their tenor – they are first and foremost packed with in-depth portraits of individuals, extracts from conversations with them, analyses of these, and references to other authorities on the subject. It is a rich and confident mix.

One chapter introduces the idea of a person with dementia as 'a semiotic subject'. In 1994 Steven and his colleague Rom Harre published a ground-breaking paper[4] in which they defined this concept as behaviour which reveals intention, which demonstrates interpretative powers, and which evaluates events and situations. This idea that people with the condition can still act in the world in various ways, and ways which are demonstrable, informs all Steven's work. Communication and its possibilities becomes the central plank in any positive philosophy of dementia, and is a major contribution to the development of caring strategies.

It is time I illustrated the unique method of Steven's presentation of his ideas. The Language chapter, from which I have already quoted, offers a vivid demonstration of the approach. It is built around an individual known as Dr B. This man was not a medical doctor but a scientist, with a strong interest in the arts. He was 68 and tests assessed him as having moderate to severe dementia. Here is an excerpt from Steve's description of their first meeting:

> Although he did grope for words at times, the tone and meaning of his sentences were clear. 'How long have you been doing this work? He asked. Suddenly, I was in the position of explaining myself to him. So I recounted to him a short history of how I came to work with AD sufferers. He asked about where I attended graduate school and when I graduated. The questions did not come fluently, for he had clear difficulty in finding the right words to use, and this resulted in protracted pauses in his words from time to time. He noted such instances by saying, 'Bear with me'. Often, about five minutes after I had answered a particular question, he asked the same question again and, once again, I answered. I told him that I was interested in learning about the remaining abilities of AD sufferers and that 'If I can work with you, maybe the results will be helpful to people.' And so began a

nine-month odyssey of cooperative research which
soon became known, in his words, as 'The Project.'
p25

This passage reveals much about the approach and its
merits. Steven is honest and straightforward in his
answers. He modifies his conversational approach to
suit his subject. He offers his partner a role in the
work, which is appreciated to the extent that he
dignifies it with a name. It contrasts markedly with
the conventional research approach of using standard
tests to elicit information, and to ignore the to-and-
fro nature of normal conversation. Here is an example
of a dialogue between Steven and Dr B about the
effects of Alzheimer's on his speech when he becomes
distracted:

Dr B	When I leave something with hiatus I think maybe I get, I wouldn't say disturbed, but it, it, it screws up the rhythm.
SRS	Oh, so if you're in the middle of thinking about something…
Dr B	Uh-huh.
SRS	And you get distracted…
Dr B	Yeah.
SRS	Then you lose what you wanted to say?
Dr B	Yeah, but um, I can, uh, wait for a little while.
SRS	Um-hum.
Dr B	And uh, I get rejuvenation, and uh, up it comes.

SRS	So there are times when you get distracted and you lose track of what you wanted to say, but if you wait a little while, it comes back?
Dr B	Ya, it'll sort of creep in.
SRS	That's really good – it's helpful to know that.
Dr B	What does it mean?
SRS	It means that you... (he interrupts)
Dr B	Is this of any value?
SRS	Are you kidding? [said in a gentle, supportive tone] Let me tell you why it's of value to me. P39

So much is happening here. First of all, it's a real conversation, with its statements, questions, answers, hesitations and interruptions. And it has a relaxed tone, so much so that Steven's 'Are you kidding?' doesn't seem out of place. Secondly, it is about a real subject they both care about and want to engage with. Thirdly, it shows Dr B's awareness, not just of his problem, but of the nature of the task they have both embarked upon: that breaking in on Steven's clarification (one of a series he is attempting) with whether what he, Dr B, is saying is of use to his companion, is of real significance. There is far more to be learned about Dr B's current preoccupation, and his communicative ability, from this short passage than from a dozen diagnostic documents.

But something else of real importance is going on here, and that is to do with the manner in which Steven interprets his role. It is the use that he makes of

'Indirect Repair' which is so significant. It is a term borrowed from linguistics, and he defines it as 'inquiring about the intention of the speaker, through the use of questions marked not by interrogatives but by intonation patterns, to the use of rephrasing what you think the speaker said and checking to see if you understood his or her meaning correctly.' The effect of this strategy is to reassure the other person and help them to retain focus and confidence.

Steven expands upon the lessons he has learned from such dialogic initiatives in the following key passage:

1   If I know that sometimes, when an AD sufferer is distracted while in the middle of a conversation, he or she might lose track of the present thought, and

2   If I know that the afflicted person might be able to retrieve the thought after a short while,

3   I would know not to interrupt the pauses during which the afflicted person was trying to retrieve the thread of conversation because

4   The interruption would serve only as yet another distraction that would exacerbate the problem and therefore

5   I would know that I should give my afflicted interlocutor more time to think before I interrupted the thought process with even so much of a question as, 'What did you want to say?' p40

What Steven has brought to the story of dementia stems from Social Constructionism. The Positioning idea, illustrated earlier in this chapter, is one of the concepts developed by that school. Briefly, the approach is concerned with Selfhood, and the various ways in which an individual responds to temporal, psychological and social factors in the environment. Insofar as a person with dementia is presented with challenges in these areas, it has an obvious contribution to make to explorative studies of communication. The means employed is equally apposite: the careful recording and analysis of verbal interactions to gain insights which can be obtained in no other way. In a personal communication, Steven expresses eloquently his humanistic philosophy, which makes him the ideal exemplar for all who wish to improve the lives of those with the condition:

> To me, speaking with people diagnosed has always been about respecting them as people and viewing them as being my teachers. It has been my job to play detective when necessary to figure out what they are trying to say... because I believe that they are always trying to communicate something. Indeed, it is exactly what we do when we encounter someone who does not speak our language but is trying to do so. We work with them to construct meaning. Active listening is the key and I believe that doing so communicates honest interest and respect and that people flourish when they feel respected and heard.

CHAPTER FIVE

The Experiencers

Christine Bryden
and
Kate Swaffer

Parallel with the development of theory and practice in psychosocial approaches to people with dementia by professionals has gone the contribution made by people with the condition themselves. This has proceeded at a slower rate, because of the necessity to convince society that they had something of value to say.

Historically, the seminal work here (not by someone with the condition) was a book *Hearing the Voice of People with Dementia: Opportunities and Obstacles* written by Malcolm Goldsmith as a result of a research project at Dementia Services Development Centre, University of Stirling.[1] Malcolm proposed that there was much to be learned from consultation, and that people with dementia had insights to share which were unavailable from any other source.

Since then a number of texts of varying quality have appeared. One of the most striking of these is *Alzheimer's From the Inside Out* by Richard Taylor.[2] However, the most consistent author in the field is Christine Bryden, with three texts available. This achievement has recently been added to by Kate Swaffer, a fellow Australian.

The first of Christine's books was *Who Will I Be When I Die*, first published in 1998 and reprinted with new material in 2012,[3] and this has been followed by *Dancing With Dementia*[4] and *Nothing About Us Without Us*.[5] (This most recent publication hardly counts, as it is a collection of powerpoints over the years, and as such is a historical document but hardly constitutes a book on the level of her other achievements.)

The aspects of her first book which made a particular impact on me when I first read it were, first of all, her vivid and detailed descriptions of how the onset of dementia affected her both physically and mentally. Although everyone with the condition has a different journey and a different pace of development, I imagine much of this would strike a chord with many individuals in a similar situation and constitutes important information for those in a supporting role.

The chapter on 'a confusion of sight and sound' is, I believe, especially valuable: it describes how easy it is for a person to experience overload in one or more of the senses, and the necessity for the person to consciously limit their involvement in situations which present problems in that area. Christine puts this cogently:

> The reason for the blank stare of many Alzheimer's patients may well be that they have been exposed to too much stimulus, so there would be little point, and indeed it may be quite counter-productive, to try to 'jolly themselves out of it' by more stimulus, whether visual or sound. p82

The second message which affected me strongly was Christine's explanation of the profound adjustment she had to make between her intellectual and emotional approach to experience. She is a woman with a very high IQ and is very self-possessed because of this (her nickname was 'I can do it'). The job she was persuaded to relinquish was demanding, and occupied her for 70–80 hours a week. Suddenly she was at home and had to adopt a limited domestic role. This is how she describes what happened:

> After years of thriving on intellectual challenges, of learning new things, of achieving change, of looking down on those at work who were not as quick in their brain gymnastics, now I have been humbled, and realise just how valueless intellect really is.

It is difficult to imagine what a dramatic turnaround this must have been for such a high-flyer. And at the time it possessed an extraordinary novelty of utterance for the reader. It forcefully presented the view that it was vitally important to engage with a person at an emotional level, and led to the discovery that the language of people with dementia can often be sensuous and imagistic rather than rational.

Thirdly, there is the mature assessment which Christine offers in her summary of just three years of rapid personal growth as a response to adapting to life-changing circumstance:

> I know that I have changed a lot already. I am more stretched out somehow, more linear, more step-by-step in my thoughts. I have lost that vibrancy, the buzz of interconnectedness, the excitement and focus I once had. I have lost the passion, the drive that once characterised me. I'm like a slow-motion version of my old self – not physically but mentally. It's not all bad, as I have more inner space in this linear mode to listen, to see, to appreciate clouds, leaves, flowers...
> I am less driven, less impatient. p62

This account was extremely valuable. First of all, it was a clear statement at a time when such statements were hard to come by. Secondly, it must be one of the first pronouncements to counter the extreme negativity that was around at the time. The awareness that there was a plus as well as a minus side to the equation and a real chance of promoting the wellbeing of people with the condition gave us a chance to counter the stigma with which we were surrounded on all sides.

Dancing With Dementia takes up where *Who Will I Be When I Die?* leaves off. This was a period of unprecedented public activity on Christine's part. It saw the founding of DASNI (Dementia Advocacy and Support Network International) in 2000, planned as an international coping with memory loss support group, and travel both within Australia and beyond, attending Alzheimer's Disease International meetings, attempting to get people with dementia onto their committees, and consultation onto their agendas. This was a major effort, and proved very taxing for someone also coping with changes in her functioning. There was, however, a major change in Christine's personal life, because she divorced her first husband and married Paul, who quickly became her support in the home and in all her political engagement.

The first part of the book chronicles these life-changing events. The rest of the text constitutes a guide for people with the condition and their carers on the needs she has identified from the many meetings and the correspondence she has had, and advice on how these can be met. Just as the first book contains essential information for all interested in dementia (largely concentrated in pages 70 to 93), so this second one has as its kernel an outline and agenda for progress in pages 89 to 166. This fulfils effectively the subtitle of the book *My Story Of Living Positively With Dementia.*

Christine's willed transformation into a spokesperson for people with the condition is impressively accomplished. It allows her to adopt 'we' in her pronouncements rather than 'I', as in the following:

> How you relate to us has a big impact on the course of the disease. You can restore our personhood, and give us a sense of being needed and valued. There is a Zulu saying that is very true 'A person is a person through others.' Give us reassurance, hugs, support, a meaning in life. p127

Christine here is close to Tom Kitwood. In the next quotation she goes even further in her identification of the qualities required of true supporters:

> As we become more emotional and less cognitive, it's the way you talk to us, not what you say, that we will remember. We know the feeling, but don't know the plot. Your smile, your laugh and your touch are what we will connect with. Empathy heals. Just take us as we are. We're still in here, in emotion and spirit, if only you could find us. p138

In these and other passages Christine is also very much on the wavelength of Steven Sabat, whom she quotes once in her book, but that is on the further subject of involvement of people with dementia in research. Where she joins forces with him is in putting communication at the centre of care. As she says:

> In my view we are not cognitively impaired but communication impaired. p117

She has much to say on other neglected aspects of dementia too:

> Depression is an excellent mimic of dementia – and for many the diagnosis is truly the beginning of the end, and a self-fulfilling prophecy. p121

> One thing that can't be overemphasised is the complex, overwhelming, often obscure and gradual, yet irregular progression of losses that occur in dementia. We need to grieve many times as each successive loss becomes apparent to us. It is hard to be continually experiencing loss and grief. p131

I must not leave this brief outline of Christine's achievements without mentioning her spirituality. As a committed Christian, she has found her religious belief a consolation and support in her travails. Without it and the constant love of her husband it is unlikely that she would have been able to aspire to the condition of *Dancing With Dementia* of her title.

Christine was diagnosed at the age of 46. Kate Swaffer was diagnosed at the age of 49, but belongs to the next generation. She has followed and built on Christine's example by speaking out and writing from the person with dementia's perspective. Her first book (we are promised others) is *What The Hell Happened To My Brain?*[6] This crude and misleading title introduces a thorough-going and highly organised text of high seriousness.

The subtitle is significant: *Living Beyond Dementia*. This is Kate's defence of it:

Living Beyond Dementia is now my preferred term to support anyone who has been diagnosed with a dementia, as a way of helping them to think about the possibility of living more positively with dementia than is currently thought possible. p186/7

Throughout a long book Kate is simultaneously attacking the status quo of society in relation to people with dementia, and proposing new ways of thinking and action. She stresses the DisAbilty agenda (her use of the word) in the following paragraph:

If the symptoms of dementia were treated as DisAbilities, the negative impact on the person, their family, and society would be far less. We would be given assistance to remain employed or to live beyond dementia, which in turn would increase our social inclusion and social equality. This would decrease the isolation, stigma and discrimination and would also reduce the negative economic impact on the person, their family and society. p186/7

The scope of Kate's book is beyond that which anyone else with dementia has attempted. She reflects upon loneliness, guilt, driving, aged care, writing and advocacy. There are two chapters (pages 83 to 102) on the perspective of the Younger Person. A lengthy discussion on grief and loss (pages 109 to 134) is particularly valuable. She has added to the vocabulary with which the subject can be discussed. BUBS is 'Back-up Brains', proposed as an alternative to 'Carers'. Her most significant innovation is the concept 'Prescribed Disengagement', which she sees as a result of how diagnoses are delivered:

> [It]sets up people with dementia to become victims or sufferers , their partners to eventually start behaving like martyrs, and to take over for the person diagnosed. It sets up people with dementia to believe there is no hope, there are no strategies to manage the symptoms of dementia, and more importantly that it's not worthwhile trying to find any. It negatively impacts self-esteem, a person's finances, relationships and the ability to see any sort of positive future. p160

Kate has been equally active as a publiciser and debater for change. This has involved her in setting up and promoting organisations which enable the voices of people to be heard. In this she was further-ing the development which had already begun in 2000. DASNI was the ground-breaker here, but it allowed family carers into membership too. Kate set up DAI (Dementia Alliance International) in 2014, which is exclusively for people with the diagnosis. The first of the national groups, on which all later ones have been modelled, was SDWG (The Scottish Dementia Working Group) in 2002. Kate was instrumental in bringing into being The Alzheimer's Australian Dementia Advisory Committee in 2014. It is impossible to overestimate the significance of this movement. For too long the history of dementia was the preserve of specialists, who only consulted family and professional carers over the nature of dementia and how its effects might be ameliorated. At last a glaring omission has begun to be rectified: the term 'Nothing About Us, Without Us' is truly being heard.

I feel I should end this chapter with a comparison of the nature of the contributions of these two remarkable individuals. The similarities of their personalities and achievements are quite striking. Pre-diagnosis both were high-achievers in terms of education and employment; both developed dementia in their forties and reflect the inadequate provision for younger people; both have obtained academic qualifications since diagnosis; both have enjoyed the support of exceptional husbands (Paul for Christine, Peter for Kate); both have been active in the political sphere (DASNI and DAI); both are highly literate and able to organise material; both have experienced slow-developing dementias, which has enabled them to make an impact over a prolonged period; and as a corollary to this latter fact, both have experienced scepticism on the part of people without the condition as to whether they have dementia or not.

What is incontrovertible is that Christine and Kate are completely untypical of the population they claim to represent. We are dealing here with two out of the 'Us' who could be involved in decision-making (currently over forty-seven million world-wide). I do not wish to suggest that many of the topics they cover, and the insights they provide, are not profoundly relevant and valuable. I do believe, however, that the history of dementia is one of people with the condition being grievously left behind. We urgently need to widen the consultation base, publish far more writings and interviews, include far more people on decision-making bodies, and get them involved in research projects.

CHAPTER SIX

The Reminiscers

Faith Gibson
and
Pam Schweitzer

For many, memory loss is what first comes to mind on thinking about dementia. And again, what comes to mind for most people when they think of memory is names, dates, people, places. But there is far more to memory than this – there is memory for emotion, habit and action. If we open our minds to the depth and complexity of memory, we can begin to explore its possibilities for enhancing the quality of life both for people with the condition and for those close to them. This initiative is called Reminiscence. The movement has succeeded in establishing life history and medical history as complementary approaches and of equal importance.

A key person during the past three decades of the Reminiscence movement has been Faith Gibson. Her quiet-spoken but authoritative presence has dominated gatherings and discussions on the subject. Born in Australia, but resident for all of that period in Northern Ireland, she became Professor of Social Work at the University of Ulster. Her books on the subject *Reminscence and Recall*, its largely rewritten and renamed fourth edition *Reminiscence and Life Story Work*[1] and *The Past in the Present*[2] are notable for their combination of intellectual rigour and user-friendliness, with their charts and checklists, practice examples and application exercises. She has, however, always viewed reminiscence as both valuable in itself and as a fruitful path into other creative interventions.

In the first part of *The Past in the Present* Faith examines memory, its dynamic and reconstructive nature, and the advantages of encouraging reminiscence in a social context. She goes on to make a fundamental claim for it in terms of preservation of the personality (of particular relevance, of course, to those with dementia):

> Regardless of age and circumstances, if one does not feel valued by others, it is difficult to value oneself. People can be reminded of their unique identity and value by recalling details of their past achievements and the esteem in which they were once held. Whether people's lives have been long or short, recalling their personal life stories reminds them and others around them of each person's singular identity and value as an individual. It helps them to continue valuing themselves, to retain control at a stage in life when events, opinions, circumstances, and other people may be eroding their independence and paying them less respect. By reminding themselves of who they used to be, they may retain a stronger sense of self in the present. p131

Chapter Three constitutes Faith's most original contribution to the literature. Here she outlines the special gift of reminiscence to staff development:

> Encouraging care staff to review their own lives can bring a heightened sense of their own uniqueness and, by implication, the uniqueness of the people whose lives they share in the course of their daily work. In a simple consciousness-raising training exercise, for example, staff could be asked to name or list three to five characteristics that make them different from other people. This provides rich material for discussions about sameness, difference, and our need

to be seen as unique individuals yet members of a group. p55

She goes on to claim:

> Through engaging in life history work, staff members glimpse the older person as he or she used to be. With new eyes, they see the long, intricate, often heroic journeys travelled by each individual. This new view radically shifts perceptions and changes relationships. Through this fresh understanding, care can be transformed. If staff members become intrigued by these intensely unique histories, then not only do their conversations become more meaningful but also their sympathy and empathy for the person – regardless of current frailty, mood and behaviour – is greatly enlarged. p56

Pam Schweitzer had a career in Theatre Education, and gradually became fascinated by Reminiscence and Oral History. In 1983 she founded the Exchange Theatre Trust in London and remained its Artistic Director until 2005. She opened the first Reminiscence Centre there in 1987, and this enthusiasm expanded into the founding of the European Reminiscence Network in 1993, with partners in 16 countries. As coordinator, an almost superhuman task for someone even with her dynamism, Pam in the succeeding years has organised conferences, seminars, festivals and training courses. In a number of these projects she has been assisted by Faith.

Pam's book on *Reminiscence Theatre*[3] has a wider remit than dementia. Her second book, written with Errolyn Bruce, *Remembering Yesterday, Caring Today*[4] however, concentrates on reminiscence with people with the condition.

This is one of the most important large-scale projects so far attempted with people with dementia, far-reaching both geographically and by ambition. The project involves groups of people with dementia and their carers meeting and revisiting their shared past experience and exploring it in a variety of ways, many involving different art-forms, objects, multi-sensory stimuli and non-verbal communication. A sizeable number of volunteers also participate. The project has been long-lasting, going through a number of phases, always evolving in an attempt to provide an inspiration to family members, empowerment for people with dementia, and generating new strategies for family and professional carers.

Faith, who has been involved in evaluating the scheme, has identified its key features as:

1   People with dementia and their caregivers participate together

2   Caregivers have some time separate from the people they care for

3   Involvement of volunteers makes the group sessions feel like normal social occasions, and volunteers also provide additional personal attention and friendship between meetings

4   Failure-free friendly groups to utilise people's strengths

5   Arts-based activities to broaden and extend non-verbal communication.[2] p242

In 2012 Catherine Ross paid a visit to the project operating at that time[5] and recorded that each group was made up of at least six pairs (person with dementia and carer), and had an artist attached to it as well as volunteers and group leaders. This made for a very intensive staff/participant ratio. She also drew attention to two other significant factors: first of all the advanced age of most of the volunteers:

> Their desire to be with, and sit alongside people with dementia is a deeply respectful starting point. They can draw effortlessly on their own memories of songs, moments, habits and styles of many years ago – something that may need explaining to those of a younger generation, and in so doing, the moment may be lost.

She also noted:

> ... The highly creative element of improvisation and intuitive risk taking led by these experienced group facilitators...

The benefits of *Remembering Yesterday, Caring Today* are various, and Pam identifies one of the most significant of them in the following passage:

> One consistent element was the carers' surprise at the extent of intact, but hitherto untapped memory revealed by the people with dementia. Knowledge of this made many carers sit up and take new notice of how they addressed their carees, what they said about them and in front of them, and how it was obviously worthwhile to make new efforts at communication by calling on retrievable past experience. Many have noted how the project has opened their eyes to how

much their person with dementia can remember and talk about, given the right stimulus and supportive environment. They have also understood that more is noted, recognised and enjoyed by their caree than can necessarily be reflected back in speech, but that participation is undoubtedly reassuring and pleasurable nevertheless. They have had fun together with their caree in ways beyond their hopes and belief; this has helped them to remember the importance of their joint past in under-pinning their ever-changing relationship in the present.[6]

Over the past five years the European Reminiscence Network has instigated an apprenticeship scheme to train performance and visual artists to work on the 'Remembering Yesterday, Caring Today' project, and this runs through European partners and has generated over 150 trained facilitators. Information on this, and much more besides, is on the website www.rememberingtogether.eu

As if the part Faith Gibson has played in the Reminiscence Movement was not sufficient achievement for one person, I have to celebrate her contribution to the wider world of dementia theory and practice made as a result of a fortuitous conjunction of a commission and her readiness to fulfil that request.

In 1999 the *Journal of Dementia Care* held conferences in the UK at which it inaugurated an annual Tom Kitwood Memorial Address. An edited version of the first address, given by Faith, was published in *JDC* under the title *Can we Risk Person-centred Communication?*[7] If I had to choose one article/essay as essential reading for all interested in the challenges dementia throws down, this would be it.

It has Faith's characteristic sense of organisation, clarity, fluency, range of reference and unflinching honesty of utterance. Its 3,000/4,000 words really deserve a chapter to themselves. Suffice it that I will illustrate its quality from a paragraph which occurs near the end. Answering the question posed by her title she writes:

> We must employ whatever power we have in the world of dementia care for this purpose. We must use our present knowledge, our skills and feelings, to communicate. We are morally obliged to continue working in extending our limited understanding, developing our embryonic skills and taming our deep anxieties. p20/24

CHAPTER SEVEN

The Artist

Anne Basting

Of the many ways in which people with dementia can be offered opportunities to maintain and even enhance their functioning, creative expression through the arts has increasingly come to be seen as a significant one. Not only does it tap in to the emotional side of people's natures, still relatively untouched by the condition, but it offers a wide choice of communicative approaches, verbal and non-verbal, and often in symbolic form, enhancing the chances to find a medium to suit the individual. Amongst its positives are: giving pleasure, providing occupation, developing a sense of flow, achievement through the process, and satisfaction if there is an end-product. One of the most important characteristics is the process of taking the personal and giving it objective form, so that experience can be looked at and evaluated. The need for this in people who are coming to terms with changes in their psyches and in their circumstances, cannot be overestimated.

Small and large projects specifically designed for people with dementia are proliferating, some traditional, others experimental in approach. It is difficult to choose one person to embody activity across the field, but I have settled on an artist, proficient in Storytelling and Drama, who has also made a contribution to the theoretical development of the subject.

Anne Basting is Professor of Theatre Arts at the University of Wisconsin, Milwaukee, USA. As an educator, scholar and artist for nearly 20 years, she has developed and researched methods for embedding the arts into long-term care, especially for people with cognitive disabilities.

One of Anne's major achievements is the Timeslips Programme.[1] This stems from a recognition that we all need to tell our own, and share others', stories, none more than the elderly experiencing memory-loss. Primarily, though, it is not about reminiscence, though memory may play a part. It harnesses imagination in the moment – stories, individual or group, just take off and soar. The process is a basic one: a prompt is provided, often a picture or an object, and a series of open-ended questions are asked; all responses are entered on a flipchart or board. These form the basis for a narrative that can go in any direction. An important rule is that no contribution offered can be rejected; all is absorbed into the whole.

Anne claims that research shows this simple formula can:

* increase the quality and quantity of interaction between staff and residents in care settings;

* improve staff and student attitudes to people with dementia;

* improve relationships between people with dementia;

* reduce medication;

* decrease distressed behaviours;

* reduce stigma

The technique has been promulgated by means of videos, manuals and training, and is now used throughout the United States and nine other countries. One activities coordinator sums up the achievement in the following words:

> I am thrilled that storytelling can be an outlet for one resident's fears and frustrations, and that it gives them a voice! It is just an incredible way to boost self-esteem and build meaningful relationships.

One of the great virtues of Anne's approach is the consistency of development that she has shown over a considerable period of time: from the original formulation of the Timeslips concept, through the development and dispersal of resources, to the Penelope Project.

Using the story from Homer's Odyssey, a team made up of staff, residents, artists and students involved a complete long-term care community in a creative enterprise. 'Finding Penelope' was the performance which resulted, but on the journey it took in discussion groups, movement exercises, visual art, storytelling and music. A two-year preparation period culminated in performances in March 2011, which over 400 people attended. All the activities took place in Luther Manor Care Facility in Milwaukee, USA.

The narrative of Penelope's rejection of 108 suitors during her husband Odysseus's absence was chosen because it was considered important to encourage the residents to feel that they were participating in an event which had a timeless aspect, even though the action had a contemporary location. The basic storyline had resonances for long-term residents because they too were playing 'a waiting game'. Anne indicates the further ideal of the project in the following words: 'Much of this work is about inviting people to be open to creativity in an environment which too often stultifies it.' She also stresses the intergenerational nature of the project.

As the play evolved the original story was turned on its head. As one of the producers states 'There are 100 Penelopes. There is a Penelope story in everyone.' so 100 suitors search for Penelope and find themselves. An actor states 'You are the ones who make the place home.' All 100 residents then chorus 'If the gods will grant us a happier old age we'll be free from our trials at last.'

The resulting book *The Penelope Project*[2] provides revealing snapshots of the process as well as practical advice for realising similar holistic initiatives in diverse settings.

Acknowledging that the project was site-specific, though it could be realised in other forms in other facilities, Anne then wanted to address the needs of the 85 per cent of older adults in America who live in their own homes, many experiencing the early stages of dementia. She has gone on to create plays which cater for this larger population.

Anne's book *Forget Memory*[3] is one of the key texts of the creativity movement. Her main thesis is that putting too great an emphasis on memory loss distorts the public view of dementia and inhibits progress towards psychosocial goals.

The two main sections of the book are devoted, first of all, to the public perception of dementia as adduced by media coverage and biases, and secondly, to positive accounts of projects in the United States which enhance people's quality of life. All the projects are arts-based and the accounts of them form the main substance of the book.

The justification for all this activity is made in two short sections at the beginning and end of the text; far more convincing are the accounts themselves, which are vividly written and provide a conclusive demonstration of the value of these initiatives. Apart from 'Timeslips' the most original of these is 'To Whom I May Concern', which provides a format and a script for those with early memory loss to act out their predicaments. Anne comments:

> With memory loss and dementia, repeating or even expressing one's thoughts or actions becomes the quintessential challenge. Family and caregivers might complain about the opposite – that people with dementia repeat themselves constantly. But the meaningful moments of exchange and self-expression can seem to evaporate in a heartbeat. Or by the time a person with memory loss pulls together thoughts and the courage to share them, the conversation has already moved so far downstream he or she doesn't bother to enter it. p87

One chapter is an evaluation of the autobiographies of people with dementia. She puts her finger on the main characteristic of Thomas de Baggio's book *Losing My Mind*:

> It seems weighted more towards the shock of his mortality at what he sees as the height of his career than a description of the actual symptoms of his condition.

And the message of the writer David Greenberger, who works with people with dementia, she sums up as:

> Be where they are. Concentrate on the sublime and ephemeral moments of a conversation. And let the brain go faster than the mouth.

In passages such as these Anne makes judgements of real cogency.

In the section of media discussions Anne comes out in favour of the film *Finding Nemo*, ostensibly nothing to do with dementia, as an enlightened portrayal of mental confusion.

Forget Memory is packed with stimulating ideas, copious notes, lists of images and stories, and descriptions of programmes. It is an invaluable resource.

Having explored multifarious ways in which people's lives can be enhanced by taking advantage of creative opportunities, in the last chapter Anne returns to the subject of memory and makes a series of points, some obvious and some less so, about the nature of this absorbing but mysterious capacity of the human. If I were to single out one of these for special emphasis it would be this:

> We must remember that memory is social, that the 'self' is relational. To forget this is to ignore one of our best 'cures' for memory loss – creating a net of social memory around a person whose individual control of memory is compromised. This doesn't mean that we should visit people more. This means that people with memory loss need to be reknit into the fabric of our lives. p161

In 2016 Anne was awarded one of the prestigious MacArthur Fellowships, for an outstanding achievement in community service and development. With her passion and dedication, we can confidently expect further impactful contributions to the creativity debate in the coming decades.

I will end with one of my favourite quotes from Anne. It is about the transformative effect which working with people with dementia can have on one's outlook on the world:[3]

> Spending time with people who have dementia has made me a more patient parent, friend, daughter, sister and wife. It's made me notice and be endlessly thankful for things like the horizon of Lake Michigan, gray storm clouds, three or four well-chosen notes on a cello, and breathing. p160

CHAPTER EIGHT

The Ethicists

Stephen Post
and
Julian Hughes

It seems likely that there is no condition more subject to disputation, apart from the existence of God, than dementia – what it is, how to prevent it, cure it and survive it. It gives rise to philosophical speculation, and every aspect of it has ethical implications. The two subjects of this chapter, Stephen Post, an American, and Julian Hughes, an Englishman, have contributed in both spheres, but I shall concentrate on their ethical work, which has shaped the debate on both sides of the Atlantic and beyond.

It is no exaggeration to say that every action or decision to withhold action in relation to our approach to a person with dementia has consequences for the person and for ourselves. And because our knowledge in this area is so scanty, right and wrong in the situations which arise are inevitably complex and provisional. Both these thinkers are aware of this at all times in their writings, which is what makes what they have to say invariably illuminating.

In 1995 Stephen Post published *The Moral Challenge of Alzheimer Disease*,[1] acknowledged by the *British Medical Journal* in 2009 as 'a medical classic of the century'. At the outset Stephen confronts the rapid rise of populations with the diagnosis and warns:

> There is potential for moral travesty or moral triumph. Because we have successfully eliminated many of the conditions that shorten the human lifespan, the thickness and thinness of our moral respect for elderly and debilitated persons takes on a new importance. p2

A radical approach which Stephen adopts is not to start with positing theories and outlining 'standards' but to take the revolutionary course of quoting extensively the words of those with the condition. He borrows a term from Habermas, a German philosopher; this is 'Discourse Ethics'. A much more pragmatic approach, he affirms, will bring insights which might elude a more formal investigation:

> Discourse ethics represents a shift away from heavy reliance on ethical theory, although without abandoning basic moral principles such as 'do no harm', beneficence, and respect for autonomy (self-determination). Such an ethics allows the process of dialogue with those who have dementia and their caregivers to define what aspects of the illness are morally important. It represents a de-emphasis on the formal professionalized canons of ethics. p17

This is just one of the ways in which dementia demands tearing up the rule-book and following new patterns of enquiry. At the same time Stephen is at pains to stress the commonality of people with and without the condition, especially in the earlier stages:

> People with dementia are meaning seeking in the way that we all are, and their struggles to make sense of loss are akin to our own. p18

If, then, as Stephen would have us do, we concentrate upon those qualities which we share with people with dementia, rather than those which divide us from them, we are led inevitably towards identifying the basic human characteristics which must be fulfilled if we are to be satisfied that we are leading moral lives. He has

articulated this more powerfully than any other commentator on dementia, and the following is a key passage
which I make no apology for quoting at length:

> Persons with cognitive disabilities need the emotional
> sense of safety and joy, and seem to reveal in the
> clearest way our universal human needs. The first
> principle of care for such persons is to reveal to them
> their value by providing attention and tenderness in
> love… The first component of love is comfort, which
> includes tenderness, calming of anxiety, and feelings of
> security based on affective closeness. It is especially
> important for the person with dementia who retains a
> sense of their lost capacities. Attachment, the second
> component of love, includes the formation of specific
> bonds that enhance a feeling of security. Other
> components of love are inclusion in social experiences,
> genuine occupation that draws on a person's abilities
> and powers, and, finally, acknowledgement of identity.
> The person with dementia, then, is part of our
> common humanity as an emotional and relational
> being and therefore must be treated with care and
> respect. Only a view of humanity that excludes
> emotion and relationality would ignore this and such
> a view would be both callous and inhumane.[2] p232/3

Stephen is not content just to state these moral principles. He sets them in a social context, and by doing so
explains why it is western societies find it so difficult
to live up to them. He expounds the theory of 'hyper-
cognitivity', which points to the emphasis on intellect
and reasoning in our education systems at the expense
of feeling and intuition. It seems that a fully functioning capitalist economy feeds on logic and downplays

the affective qualities. Since intellectual capacity tends to be undermined by dementia, though feeling-states remain, and those around the person lack expertise in the latter capacities, there is an inevitable mis-match between the caring attitudes desired and those on offer.

He explores the consequences of this in the following paragraph:

> In our own hypercognitive culture, currently so captivated by eugenic images of human perfection both physical and mental, it is easy to think that people with dementia simply do not count morally; that is, they lack any moral significance. We divide 'them' from 'us', drawing a line between the rational and the less rational, the unforgetful and the most forgetful, thereby exposing people with dementia to a vulnerability manifest in disregard of their remaining capacities, subjectivity and well-being. Abuse and neglect of people with dementia is a perennial tendency.[1] p32

Despite his misgivings on this front, Stephen goes on to suggest an innovative approach to those people with dementia nearing the end of their lives; it is a kind of special hospice for those with the condition, based on the principle of 'being with' rather than 'doing to'. Alongside any necessary medical treatments, he proposes a counselling approach offered with the utmost sensitivity, and a raft of arts activities alongside haptic (touch) and relaxation sessions.

One of the most striking embodiments of Stephen's philosophy is contained in the final sentence of his contribution to the edited book already excerpted from:

> Equal regard based on the cognitive, emotional, relational, and symbolic-expressive aspects of persons with dementia (including advanced dementia) lead me to reject the notion 'I think, therefore I am' and replace it with the less arrogant 'I feel and relate, and therefore I am'.[2] p233

Stephen Post is Professor of Bioethics in the Case School of Medicine, Case Western Reserve University, USA. Julian Hughes was for many years a consultant in old age psychiatry at North Tyneside General Hospital, and an Honorary Clinical Senior Lecturer at the Institute for Ageing and Health in the University of Newcastle, UK. Julian has written very extensively on ethical issues, often in collaborative enterprises. One such is the book, described as a 'practice guide', *Ethical Issues in Dementia Care: Making Difficult Decisions*, co-authored with Clive Baldwin.[3] This text is remarkable for its clarity in both construction and expression, in an area notable for its pitfalls. It is also full of case-examples, whether real or imaginary, and these illuminate what might otherwise appear abstractions.

Julian and Clive adopt a rather different approach from Stephen. This is an exposition of the field, and as such they are less interested in making judgements or proposing theories than painstakingly elucidating ideas and approaches already identified. They do not, however, avoid acknowledging that decision-making in this area is 'messy'. By this they mean that whatever ethical framework is adopted, real-life situations throw the individual into making decisions which are provisional, and may indeed prove to have been imperfect.

That said, numerous theories and ideas are explored in this text, and some judgements made, One is that conscience alone is a poor guide to action. Another is that quality of life is very difficult to define because it is constituted of so many different domains. 'Discourse Ethics' echoes the use by Stephen of the term, but Julian and Clive offer the proviso:

> Older people have gradually been placed in a position, reflecting societal and political pressures, where they have no real choice. They may have to accept long-term care because there is no political will to provide alternatives. p103–4

'Narrative Ethics' is also covered here, which is defined as:

> The right decision will emerge from a correct understanding of the person's story and where they are situated in this co-created history. p106

An advantage of this latter concept is that it well reflects the complexities of people's lives, both within the family and outside it. It also assists with meeting the demands of end-of-life issues.

The book ends with a consideration of 'patterns of practice', an attempt to enumerate all the different ways of approaching issues, and a plea for openness in relation to ethical decisions, rather than inflexible rule-making.

Julian occupies an unusual position in the history of dementia. It is impossible to pigeonhole him. I suppose this is a way of saying that he is the most notable polymath of the subject. He has written a book *Alzheimer's and Other Dementias*,[4] which is probably the best potted version of the medical side of things. The co-edited contributed volume *Dementia: Mind, Meaning and Person* addresses philosophical, psychological and social aspects of the subject. Like Stephen, he is interested in end-of-life issues, and has written a book about it *Palliative Care in Severe Dementia*,[5] and as a thinker his most extended meditation on a spectrum of issues is *Thinking Through Dementia*,[6] a volume of almost 300 densely argued pages. That there are more references in the Index to Wittgenstein than any other person attests to Julian's philosophical credentials, but, of course, ethical considerations earn their place.

The book critiques biomedical, neuropsychological and social constructionist perspectives, and attempts a synthesis of common attributes. Julian also adopts the widest possible approach to ethical issues. For example, he draws attention to decision-making in relation to resources for treatment and research, and within the research sphere decisions whether money should be allocated towards searching for a cure or developing psychological approaches. A major point he makes is in relation to facts, which on the surface would appear to be value-free, but he claims that this is not so:

> It is not just that facts reflect values in the sense that values emerge from them in their interpretation. The second possibility I wish to consider is that facts themselves are value-laden: facts presuppose values. p11

He goes on to apply this precept to diagnosis, where he draws attention to the way dementia:

> is seen as an 'organic' condition where the facts of brain pathology obscure the surrounding evaluative considerations. p12

These ideas are promoted at the outset. At the end of his prolonged examination of the many facets of his subject, Julian offers this provocative observation:

> The tendency for older people to be marginalised or discriminated against, the tendency for their standing as selves to be undermined, the possibility for alienation from themselves, these are all political matters. The cry of solidarity and the demand for citizenship should be our response to the undermining of the human rights of large parts of our societies worldwide simply because they are aging and, in particular, because of dementia. p269

CHAPTER NINE

The Unifier

Peter Whitehouse

I began this attempt to identify a narrative of the deeply puzzling phenomenon of dementia with Alois Alzheimer, a man who, seemingly unwittingly, invented a health category, and my final choice is that of someone who embodies in his own personal journey the dilemmas with which that construct has presented us.

Peter Whitehouse, born in London, but currently Professor of Neurology at Case Western Reserve University Ohio, Strategic Advisor in Innovation at Baycrest Health Center, and Professor of Medicine at the Institute of Life Course and Ageing at the University of Toronto, began his career as a convinced clinician, a doctor who in his practice fully subscribed to the disease model, and in his research accepted the funding of drug companies to promulgate the message. Now he is an outspoken critic of that approach, and a leading proponent of psychosocial strategies.

The title of his book, published in 2008, *The Myth of Alzheimer's: What You Aren't Being Told About Today's Most Dreaded Diagnosis* sets the tone, and early on in the text he explains his motivation for writing it in the following words:

> to empower readers to stand up to the dominant, stigmatizing biological myth of Alzheimer's that scientists like myself, with more than a little help from the drug companies and others with personal and financial interests, have unleashed on individual lives, and to reframe the way we know and experience our aging selves. p43

Peter devotes a chapter to the life of Alois, and tells it in very much the same way as I have, though in greater detail. He brings out the almost coincidental way in which the diagnosis was made, and includes a significant quote from Alois which seems to have been overlooked by later commentators: *There is no tenable reason to consider my cases as caused by a specific disease process.*

Peter rejects the idea that Alzheimer's is a unique medical condition, which allows him to phrase the basic challenge, the central question to be considered, as:

> Should biomedical disease labels with frightening cultural meanings be used to describe a condition that might be considered variable human aging? p39

An alternative scenario of the history of dementia than the one I have chosen to present would have chronicled the various discoveries and the products developed to meet the challenges identified. Being qualified to do this, and wanting to give a balanced picture, Peter offers an account, though he is at pains to emphasise how little has been achieved in this area, despite the large sums expended.

Another plot for the story could have been a historical perspective of the development of organizations devoted to the condition, especially the Alzheimer Societies, both national and international, and their successes in setting the agendas in both spheres.

Peter covers both of these aspects, and the strong links that have been developed between them, particularly the way much of the money raised by the latter has helped to fund the research of the former. He is highly critical of the way they have accomplished the medicalization of ageing:

> The Alzheimer's movement is a march-to-progress juggernaut: Give us enough time, people and money, the line goes, and we will fix it. But after 30 years of research, and tens of billions of dollars spent, we're not even close. In fact, our expensive genetic tests and neuroimaging devices have actually caused us to drift deeper into confusion and little closer to finding a cure. We are giving people false hope.

Later in the same key paragraph he presents, in essence, his positive proposal for remedying the situation:

> Shouldn't we begin to consider reallocating some of our resources into other avenues, for example investing in educating people as to the preventive (behavioural) measures we can all take over the course of our life spans to avoid damage to our brains, and developing alternative therapies such as narrative-based, music and touch interventions, or, on developing innovative caregiving practices for the patients and families who are adapting to memory challenges? p40

Elsewhere in the text he adds to this non-medical prescription 'the rhythms of the body and its functions', opportunities to improve our non-verbal skills and caring responses, enjoy more sensory experiences, and discover 'a wellspring of energy and compassion that is more healing than any pharmaceutical pill'. p106

Peter's, we see here, is a lifelong holistic solution to the problems created by the prolongation of our lifespan and its consequent effects on brain and body. He encourages us to engage in the process of reconsidering Alzheimer's, which in turn will lead to reconsidering ageing, which in turn will lead to reconsidering what constitutes being human.

Instead of acceding to the disease model he prefers to see memory loss and related features becoming increasingly normalised as we grow older. The logical end-result of this process if the present trajectory continues is that we will reach a point where everyone could develop the condition. Given the present situation, however, he is concerned with the social effects of the focus on the biological approach, and the widespread fears that stigma creates. It is not surprising, therefore, that his view of the rush to diagnosis is one of alarm and distrust:

> Every time a diagnosis of Alzheimer's is made, we
> must remember that it can be as socially destructive as
> it is scientifically uncertain. p77

Peter is not just an apologist for alternative approaches, however; he has made an important contribution to one of the areas listed above: that of education. He and his wife Cathy founded an intergenerational school in Cleveland, Ohio. This institution has been rewarded with recognition by state, regional and local authorities. The emphasis is on lifelong learning and the curriculum emphasises reading, computing and gardening. The learning experiences of six to twelve year olds is shared with elders, many of whom are living with dementia. Within the school there is a Shaker Nature

Centre, which in 2015 won the Rachel Carson Sense of Wonder Prize presented by the Environmental Protection Agency for Multimedia Narratives.

Here is a story from the school. One member of staff won the school's Volunteer of the Year award. When she stepped up to receive the prize she asked a friend 'Why am I getting this award?' 'Because you volunteer and come here ever week, and the children love you' was the reply she received. 'Do I?' she asked. She could not remember the service she gave, yet she was an indispensable member of the team.

Peter sums up the achievement in the following words:

> In The Intergenerational School we are demonstrating
> that a different model of public education can not
> only provide better learning for children, but can also
> create opportunities for older adults to contribute in a
> personal way to the future of their communities, share
> their collective wisdom, and stay cognitively vital in
> the process. p146

Peter devotes chapters to discussing the various drugs which have been developed, their potency and their side-effects, and also mounts a critique of genetics and molecular medicine. He believes that there is a great deal of what he describes as 'overpromising' in this area, and that what was initially perceived as offering hopes of greater personalising of medicine is actually leading to its opposite: by concentrating on genetic blueprints rather than the likely multiple causes of dementia the whole person is being side-lined yet again through biomedical bias.

Because his book is intended for the ordinary reader, Peter devotes his final chapters to what he calls 'A New Model for Brain Aging'. This consists of valuable advice on how to get the best out of your doctor, asserting yourself in medical situations, and contributing to research. He offers especial guidance on how to receive a diagnosis. All this contains exceptionally useful information from a reliable source. He deals with diet and exercise, avoiding stress and practising cognitive stimulation. He recommends participating in community activities wherever possible. In a ringing mantra he sums up all this as 'Making a Profession out of Prevention'.

In various contexts throughout his book Peter brings up the idea of storytelling as a fundamental human activity. In his final chapter he commends both Reminiscence (Chapter Six) and Timeslips (Chapter Seven) as having contributions to make to quality of life. But he would encourage us to recognise and value story processes as essential to making sense of our experiences (and I would wish to add that that, of course, has been my motivation in trying to gain perspective on dementia in this book). He recommends Life-Book-making, in which we record our challenges and achievements, and demonstrate our awareness of growth and development as a lifelong process. He wittily characterises his own narrative progression as that of from Brain-Bank to Story-Bank. There is indeed a project he has set up in Ohio under the latter name to collect the health experiences of individuals.

In his Epilogue Peter quotes a 90-year-old philosopher he met in Norway who told him the principle he
lived by was 'Think Like a Mountain'. At first this
concept puzzles him. But then he realises that the
mountain has a secure base on which it is founded, its
surface shows the results of ageing, and it appears to
be reaching for the sky. As humans we can identify
with these characteristics, but we also have creativity
which we can harness to modify our environment.

In a sense I see Peter as the Unifier in the history of
dementia. Of course he's also the Iconoclast, the
dismantler of the dominance of the medical model.
Singlehandedly he has mounted a distinctive attack on
the largely barren field of biological research, and is
the upholder of a broader, more humane vision of how
we might approach the subject. He has capitalised on
the Kitwood legacy, incorporating the advances made
by those featured in my chapters, and others who
have made a contribution. He has drawn together the
psychosocial threads to make a coherent garment for
us all to wear.

Has Dementia a Future?

Over the past nine chapters I have attempted to chart a history of dementia. It is no doubt a partial and biased account. It is difficult to obtain perspective on a subject which is growing and changing before our eyes. And although I am not a specialist or carer or person with the condition but a writer, and therefore might be considered as an objective commentator, through my direct work with people with dementia over the past quarter of a century, and the books I have written which have come out of that experience, I could be considered to have played a small part in the picture I have painted. Readers must bear this in mind in relation to what they have read and to what follows.

The title of this postscript asks a provocative question. Because of where we are in the story, with numbers of people diagnosed worldwide increasing, alongside provision of services and the expenditure on research, the short-term answer has to be a confident yes. But what about the longer view – will the word 'dementia' still be in use, say, 50 years from now? And, even more controversially, will the condition we refer to by it still exist in its present form or have been eradicated or morphed into something else?

To take the language first, there is surely a case for getting rid of a word which stands for, as Peter White-house puts it, 'today's most dreaded diagnosis' (White-house 2008)? There have been various attempts to change the associations by changing the terminology. Modifying a concept has to be a long-term aim rather than an instant achievement. I suspect that it takes time for people's memories to adjust, maybe a generation to pass? They've tried it in Japan, and it will be interesting to see if the new descriptor catches on. It used to be *chihou*, translated as 'losing your mind, stupid' and is now *ninchishou* which means 'awareness of cognitive symptoms'. 'What's in a name?' you may ask. Obviously a great deal, or the Japanese government wouldn't have put so much money into this project. At least the new term was a result of a public consultation.

The second aspect is whether the condition will have been dropped or absorbed into something else. By this I do not mean to suggest, as the Alzheimer's Societies do, that a cure will be found if only we give them enough money. That is either ridiculous or duplicitous or both. No, I mean that either a whole series of advances may have been made, medically and socially, so that the effects of the condition have been rendered harmless and acceptable. That is surely possible. We would, of course, have to stop frightening people by using the terminology of warfare – not fighting the phenomenon but collaborating with it. I know, that is a big ask, and could take decades.

But now I should like to suggest something even more radical, something which would involve a sea-change in attitudes, nothing less than a change in our world-picture and the way society thinks and is organised.

There is an ancient document called the 'Mappa Mundi' in Hereford Cathedral in the UK. This extraordinary piece of work is a plan of the world as it appeared to the mediaeval mind. It is a mixture of topography, history, natural history, mythology, religion and cosmology. It bears little relation to our current concept of the world, or even our conventional view of a map. We now see topography as the predominant feature, and confine other aspects to maps which concentrate on individual categories (political, climatic, vegetational etc.). Our topographical maps are now amazingly detailed: we can even gain accurate impressions of the land beneath the seas, for example, and the currents which pass through them. No doubt those who proudly designed the 'Mappa Mundi' were convinced that their picture was comprehensive and accurate, whilst in reality it was nothing of the kind.

More recently LN Fowler in the mid-19th century in the US marketed a bust of a head labelled with 'powers' and 'organs'. Around the back of the cranium were the following words:

> For thirty years I have studied crania and living heads from all parts of the world and have found in every instance there is a perfect correspondence between the conformation of an individual and his known characteristics.

Parts of the brain were labelled 'Moral', 'Aspiring', 'Domestic', 'Reflective', 'Perceptive' and 'Self-Reflective'. This formed a contribution to a movement initiated earlier by Gall in Vienna and titled 'Phrenology'. It was very influential at the time, but it was, if you'll pardon the pun, an attempt which proved completely 'wrong-headed'!

Both these initiatives, convincing in their day, were absurdly over-ambitious in their attempts to construct systems out of physical and other data. Might there be some correspondence between the 'Mappa Mundi' and 'Phrenology' views of world and brain on the one hand, and our contemporary view of dementia on the other? If we are honest we have to admit that our knowledge in this area is so imperfect that it may be totally misguided. Approaching it from the physical side, which has largely dominated the research community up to the present, may be viewing through the wrong end of the telescope? Perhaps the tentative attempts of most of those featured in these chapters may prove more fruitful in the long run? And there are aspects, also of a psychosocial nature, which I have not touched on because currently they have not found their leaders, aspects such as counselling (both individual and group), and spirituality, which may lead to insights of real potency which can help us to a new understanding and mapping.

I cannot claim to have other than glimmerings of where the dementia story may take us next. What I am certain of, though, is that the one presented to us by the self-styled gurus (no names here, and they receive no mentions in this book), the organisations set up to promote care and research, and the media which present watered-down or distorted versions of this story, is seriously inadequate. To adopt a literary metaphor, we are offered a sketch, when what we are dealing with is a book of the proportions and intricacy of a novel.

So my personal answer to the question posed at the outset is: no, I don't think dementia, as at present conceived, or mis-conceived, has a future. Something as little understood, as fumblingly diagnosed, as inhumanely treated, does not deserve prolongation. But we will be stuck with it if we don't do something about ourselves, our economic, political and social institutions – in short, our whole way of life. We have the dementia we deserve: maybe we have created it out of a combination of ignorance and greed, out of following the wrong star. If we can change course in time and concentrate on creating compassionate integrated societies we could see it wither on the vine. I am living in hope that this story will have a happy ending.

1906   Frau D dies – Alzheimer delivers
                        three-page paper identifying a
                        distinctive pathology, suggesting
                        the existence of a form of
                        dementia that will come to be
                        known as Alzheimer's disease.

1910   Kraepelin publishes on
                        subdivision of senile dementia in
                        3rd edition of Psychiatrie –
                        'Alzheimer's disease'

1920   'Dementia' starts to be used for
                        what is now understood as
                        schizophrenia and senile dementia

1929–1932   Three investigators identified
                        what appeared to be familial
                        patterns of inheritance in two
                        generations: Flügel, Schottky,
                        Lowenberg

1933 Gellerstedt   Over 80 per cent of all
                        non-demented individuals over
                        age 65 had some senile plaques
                        and tangles – complicating the
                        diagnosis

1979   Alzheimer Association founded
                        (as Alzheimer Disease and Related
                        Diseases Association)

1980   Alzheimer's included in the DSM

1983	Pam Schweitzer founds the Age Exchange Theatre Trust
1986	Age Concern Scotland chooses dementia as its theme
1987	First Reminiscence Centre is opened in London
1989	Dementia Services Development Centre at University of Stirling founded
1992	Alzheimer's Research Trust founded
1993	European Reminiscence Network founded
1994	Mary Marshall directs session on 'The Experience of Dementia' – the first forum of its kind in the world
1994	Ronald Reagan announces diagnosis of Alzheimer's
1995	*The Moral Challenge of Alzheimer Disease* by Stephen Post published
1997	*Dementia Reconsidered: the person comes first* by Tom Kitwood
1998	*Who Will I Be When I Die?* By Christine Bryden published

1999	Inaugural Tom Kitwood Memorial Address given by Faith Gibson at the JDC conference
2000	Dementia Advocacy and Support Network International founded
2000	The Intergenerational School founded
2001	Steven Sabat publishes *The Experience of Alzheimer's Disease*
2002	Iris Murdoch Centre at University of Stirling opened – the first purpose-built dementia-friendly building
2005	Mary Marshall publishes *Perspectives on Rehabilitation and Dementia*
2008	*The Myth of Alzheimer's: What You Aren't Being Told About Today's Most Dreaded Diagnosis* by Peter Whitehouse published
2011	*Finding Penelope* performed in Luther Manor Care Facility, Milwaukee USA
2014	The Alzheimer's Australian Dementia Advisory Committee founded (by Kate Swaffer)

There are those who will say that my book is so biased as to be a distortion of the truth.

To them I would answer that dementia is a subject where 'the truth' is something in short supply, and 'my truth' has as much right to its existence as any other.

Moreover, mine is a narrative of modest advances, and has no large expensive failures to apologise for.

It is by no means a complete picture, and doesn't claim to be. It doesn't seek to denigrate those who are currently beavering away throughout the world in honest attempts to find 'a cure', or rather a multiple set of medical breakthroughs.

Nor does it undervalue the work of those who are in search of preventive measures, such as diet, exercise and intellectual stimulation; these are important components of the positive picture to which it aspires to belong.

What this book does claim, though, is that it favours an initiative which puts actions in the hands of people with dementia and their supporters. Nature, we are told, abhors a vacuum, and a diagnosis followed by a period of depressive helplessness must be avoided. Practical steps have been proposed and taken by my chosen champions, and foundations have been laid, which I believe are sound and sensible, for us all to build upon.

Counselling is a subject which is clearly applicable to dementia, yet a movement to establish it has hardly got off the ground. This is partly due to the undue emphasis that has been placed on the medical aspects of the condition, which this book has set out to remedy, and the consequent lack of emphasis on what is, admittedly, an expensive option. Nevertheless, the lack of interest in a subject which has so much to offer to the individual, and could yield fresh insights into the condition, is nothing less than shameful.

The book I would recommend is *Person-Centred Counselling for People with Dementia: Making Sense of Self* (Jessica Kingsley Publications) by Danuta Lipinska. Early in the book she says:

> At the heart of my endeavour is my wish to combine a particular 'way of being' a counsellor and plant it firmly within the person-centred approach to dementia care, placing the experiential within the practical.

Her philosophy is based firmly upon that of Carl Rogers, and she has read her Kitwood closely. She is particularly good on process, and her text is illuminated by many anecdotes. She does not shirk the spiritual implications of this work. Reading her book shows us how much we are missing by bypassing the in depth approaches.

Danuta has a new book out from Jessica Kingsley Publications towards the end of 2017. It is called *Dementia, Sex and Wellbeing: Strange Bedfellows.*

* * *

In choosing those individuals to focus on in my chapters I am conscious that I have omitted any family carer, and that means a whole swathe of personal narratives. I have to confess that, despite their emotionalism, many of them leave me cold: there is only so much I can take of whining negativity. Sally Magnusson's *Where Memories Go: why dementia changes everything* is something else. Despite being over-long and over-ambitious it gets the main thing right: it gives a balanced view of the condition and coping with it as a carer.

She does have her moans, and they are fully justified:

> Older people take their lives into their hands when they enter any hospital. Perhaps a notice at every hospital entrance might help: 'STAY OUT' it would say 'Entering may endanger your health'.

At the same time the book contains passages such as the following:

> Such a precious thing, a thought expressed. My sisters and I are becoming adept at easing them into the world, like midwives.

The key chapters are those on community, identity and music. Her enthusiasm for the last has lead to her establishing the charity 'Playlist for Life' (www.playlistforlife.org.uk)

* * *

Sometimes true knowledge of a subject comes not from those who spend a lifetime studying it, but a creative artist who temporarily turns the searchlight beam of their emotional intelligence upon it, so we must not neglect the novelist who, throughout an extended narrative, can develop an interpretation. Such a writer is the American Elizabeth Cohen.

In her book *The House on Beartown Road* (Random House) she tells the story of an unusual threesome. There's Elizabeth the mother, her young daughter Ava, and her ageing father who has dementia. Elizabeth's husband has walked out on her. The plot is based on how they all shake down together after a rocky start. Relationships and language are common themes. Much of the playfulness and pathos come from the resemblances and dissimilarities of the very young and the very old. It's an easy read, and full of genuinely humorous situations, often caused by misunderstandings.

The messages are often profound, however. In one of her serious moments the author offers one of my favourite quotations:

> I think that a sense of humour must be hidden in a box very deep in the brain, where diseases have to search for it. Maybe this is an evolutionary tactic, to keep people going.

I believe this book has a basis in fact, which must be what gives it its wonderful authenticity.

* * *

The majority of people with the diagnosis in the West remain in their own homes, though care establishments loom large in the public mind, either through the personal or financial losses involved. G. Allen Power in his book *Dementia Beyond Drugs: Changing the culture of care* (Health Professions Press) addresses most of the major issues head on. He is a medical doctor, and so his polemic overthrowing the panoply of arguments for antipsychotics carries special force. He is writing from within the care home system and bolsters his arguments with copious real life situations and stories. Like Peter Whitehouse he attacks the unholy alliance between the drugs companies and the dementia charities, and he speculates what the effect would be if wellness rather than illness was the raison d'etre of the system. He is an advocate of the 'Eden Alternative' model (www.edenalt.org). His radical views include the abolition of dementia-specific units.

In common with other advocates of psychosocial approaches, Dr Power sees language as a tool for change:

> If the biomedical model is inadequate, then terminology rooted in the biomedical view of dementia must be replaced with words that reflect a person-directed, experiential view.

* * *

Lastly, 17 years since his first, Steven Sabat has a new book on the stocks. *Alzheimer's Disease and Dementia: What Everyone Needs to Know* (Oxford University Press) is expected early in 2018. Amongst the positive characteristics it is expected to deliver are: strengths of the person with the condition, and how the caregiver can identify these; how people diagnosed cope with this experience, as well as their sense of self and the social world; and how the caregiver can avoid dysfunctional treatment, and also avoid unwittingly interpreting normal actions as pathological. It should provide a new benchmark for enlightened approaches.

Chapter One

1   Hoff P (1991) Alzheimer's and his time. In
    Berrios GB & Freeman HL, eds. *Alzheimer's and
    the Dementias*. London: Royal Society of
    Medicine Services, 29–56.

2   Maher BA (1970) *Principles of Psychopathology*.
    New York: McGraw Hill.

3   Henderson AS (1983) *The Coming Epidemic of
    Dementia*. Australian and New Zealand Journal
    of Psychiatry 17 (2) 117–127.

4   Woods RT (1989) *Alzheimer's Disease: Coping
    with a Living Death*. London: Souvenir Press.

5   Alzheimer A (1977) A unique illness involving
    the cerebral cortex. In DA Rottenberg and FH
    Hochberg (eds) *Neurological Classics in Modern
    Translation*. New York: Hafner Press.

6   Breuer J and Freud S (1955) Studies on hysteria.
    in J Strachey (ed) *Studies in Hysteria. The
    standard edition of the Complete Psychological
    Works of Sigmund Freud*. Volume 2. London:
    The Hogarth Press. First published 1895.

7   Cheston R, Bender M (1999) *Understanding
    Dementia: The Man with the Worried Eyes*.
    London: Jessica Kingsley Publishers, 22–45.

8   Kitwood T (1997) *Dementia Reconsidered: the
    person comes first*. Buckingham: Open University
    Press, 35.

Chapter Two

1   Kitwood T (1970) *What is Human?*. Inter-Varsity Press.

2   Kitwood T (1997) *Dementia Reconsidered: the person comes first*. Buckingham: Open University Press.

3   Baldwin C & Capstick A (2007) *Tom Kitwood on Dementia: A Reader and Critical Commentary*. Maidenhead: Open University Press.

Chapter Three

1   Marshall M (1997) *State of the Art in Dementia Care* London: Centre for Policy on Ageing p13

2   Marshall M (1997) Therapeutic Design for People with Dementia in Hunter S ed. in *Dementia: Challenges and New Directions* London: Jessica Kingsley Publishers p181

3   Judd S, Phippen P, Marshall M. eds. (1998) *Design for Dementia* (1998) London: Hawker.

4   Marshall M (2010) *Designing Balconies, Roof Terraces and Roof Gardens for People with Dementia*. Scotland: University of Stirling.

5   Pollock A, Marshall M (2012) *Designing Outdoor Spaces for People with Dementia*. University of Stirling/Hammond Care.

6   Marshall M, Gilliard J (2014) *Creating Culturally Appropriate Outside Spaces and Experiences for People with Dementia: Using Nature and the Outdoors in Person-centred Care*. London: Hawker.

7   Marshall M (2005) Risk and Choice *Journal of Dementia Care* 13(3)5
8   Marshall M ed. (2005) *Perspectives on Rehabilitation and Dementia*. London: Jessica Kingsley Publishers p13
9   Marshall M (2000) *ASTRID: A Social and Technological Response to Meeting the Needs of Individuals with Dementia and their Carers*. London: Hawker Publications.
10   Marshall M (ed), ((2003) *Food, Glorious Food: perspectives on food and dementia*. London: Hawker Publications.
11   Gilliard J, Marshall M (eds) (2010) *Time For Dementia: A collection of writings on the meanings of time and dementia* (2010) London: Hawker Publications p5
12   Gilliard J, Marshall M (eds) (2012) *Fresh Air On My Face: Transforming the Quality of Life For People With Dementia Through Contact With the Natural World* (2012) London: Jessica Kingsley Publishers p148

Chapter Four

1   Sabat R S (2001) *The Experience of Alzheimer's Disease: Life Through a Tangled Veil*. London: Blackwell.
2   Luria A R (1987) *The Mind of a Mnemorist* Cambridge, Massachusetts: Harvard University Press.
3   Harre R, van Langenhove L (1999) *Positioning Theory* Oxford: Blackwell.

4 Sabat R, Harre R (1994) The Alzheimer's
   Disease Sufferer as a Semiotic Subject.
   Philosophy, Psychiatry, Psychology 1 145–60

Chapter Five

1 Goldsmith M (1996) *Hearing the Voice of People
   with Dementia: Opportunities and Obstacles.*
   London: Jessica Kingsley Publishers

2 Taylor R (2008) *Alzheimer's From the Inside
   Out.* Baltimore: Health Professions Press

3 Bryden C (2012) *Who Will I Be When I Die?*
   London: Jessica Kingsley Publishers

4 Bryden C (2006) *Dancing With Dementia: My
   Story of Living Positively With Dementia.*
   London: Jessica Kingsley Publications

5 Bryden C (2016) *Nothing About Us, Without Us:
   20 Years of Dementia Advocacy.* London: Jessica
   Kingsley Publications

6 Swaffer K (2016) *What the Hell Happened to
   My Brain? Living Beyond Dementia.* London:
   Jessica Kingsley Publications

Chapter Six

1 Gibson F (2011) *Reminiscence and Life Story
   Work: A Practice Guide.* London: Jessica
   Kingsley Publishers

2 Gibson F (2004) *The Past in the Present: Using
   Reminiscence in Health and Social Care.*
   Baltimore: Health Professions Press

3 Schweitzer P (2006) *Reminiscence Theatre:*

Making Theatre From Memories. London: Jessica Kingsley Publishers

4   Schweitzer P, Bruce E (2006) *Remembering Yesterday, Caring Today: Reminiscence in Dementia Care*. London: Jessica Kingsley Publishers

5   Ross C (2012) Remembering Together. *Journal of Dementia Care* 20(3)22–24

6   Schweitzer P (1999) Remembering Yesterday: a European Perspective. *Journal of Dementia Care* 7(1)16–21

7   Gibson F (1999) Can We Risk Person-centred Care? *Journal of Dementia Care* 7(5) 20–24

Chapter Seven

1   Timeslips www.timeslips.org

2   Basting A, Towey M, Rose E (2016) *The Penelope Project: An Arts-Based Odyssey to Change Elder Care*. Iowa City: Iowa University Press

3   Basting A (2009) *Forget Memory: Creating Better Lives for People with Dementia*. Baltimore: The Johns Hopkins University Press

Chapter Eight

1   Post S G (1995) *The Moral Challenge of Alzheimer's Disease*. Baltimore: The Johns Hopkins University Press

2   Hughes J C, Louw S J, Sabat S R (2006) *Dementia: Mind, Meaning and the Person*. Oxford: Oxford University Press

3   Hughes J C, Baldwin C (2006) *Ethical Issues in Dementia Care: Making Difficult Decisions.* London: Jessica Kingsley Publications
4   Hughes J C (2011) *Alzheimer's and Other Dementias.* Oxford: Oxford University Press
5   Hughes J C (2005) *Palliative Care in Severe Dementia.* New York: Lippincott
6   Hughes J C (2011) *Thinking Through Dementia.* Oxford: Oxford University Press

Chapter Nine
1   Whitehouse P J, George D (2008) *The Myth of Alzheimer's: What You Aren't Being Told About Today's Most Dreaded Diagnosis.* New York: St Martin's Press

ALOIS ALZHEIMER

Dr Aloysius 'Alois' Alzheimer (German: 14 June 1864 – 19 December 1915) was a German psychiatrist and neuropathologist and a colleague of Emil Kraepelin. Alzheimer is credited with identifying the first published case of 'presenile dementia', which Kraepelin would later identify as Alzheimer's disease.

TOM KITWOOD

Professor Thomas Kitwood (Boston, Lincolnshire: 16 February 137 – 1 November 1998) was a pioneer in dementia care. He was Senior Lecturer in Psychology at Bradford University 1984–98, and named Alois Alzheimer Professor of Psychogerontology in 1998. His innovative research challenged the 'old culture of care' in favour of understanding the standpoint of the person with dementia. His major innovation to achieve this goal was Dementia Care Mapping, a method for observational evaluation of the quality of care that is provided in formal settings, such as care homes, or home care providers. His book is *Dementia Reconsidered* (1997).

MARY MARSHALL

Mary Marshall is Hon. Professor at the University of Edinburgh and Professor Emeritus at the University of Stirling, where she was the director of the Dementia Services Development Centre between 1989 and 2005. Beginning her career as a social worker for older people, she has worked in dementia care for over 30 years. She is now associate consultant with the Dementia Centre, UK. She is a prolific author and lecturer, specialising in dementia design and care.

STEVEN SABAT

Professor Steven R. Sabat earned his doctorate at the City University of New York, where he specialized in Neuropsychology. His research involves the cognitive and social abilities of people with Alzheimer's disease, the subjective experience of having the disease, and the ways in which communication between those diagnosed and their caregivers may be enhanced. His publications include *The Experience of Alzheimer's Disease: Life Through a Tangled Veil* (Blackwell, 2001) and his co-edited book, *Dementia: Mind, Meaning, and the Person* (Oxford University Press, 2006).

CHRISTINE BRYDEN

Christine Bryden is the author of *Who Will I Be When I Die?* (1998) and *Dancing with Dementia* (2006) and is a passionate advocate for people with dementia. Before her diagnosis in 1995, she was a biochemist and a science publisher. As a senior executive in the Australian public service, she was awarded the Public Service Medal for her outstanding service to science and technology. *Who Will I Be When I Die?* recounts the emotional rollercoaster she experienced after her diagnosis.

KATE SWAFFER

Kate Swaffer is a poet, blogger, author and speaker. Since her dementia diagnosis in 2008, she has completed three degrees and is now a PhD student at the University of Wollongong. She is an advocate and activist for aged and dementia care. With Dementia Alliance International, Kate is a voice for 47.5 million people worldwide living with dementia. She was the first person with dementia to be a keynote speaker at a World Health Organisation conference. Her book is *What the Hell Happened to My Brain?* (2016)

FAITH GIBSON

Faith Gibson OBE is Emeritus Professor of Social
Work at the University of Ulster, Northern Ireland.
She trained as a social worker and teacher in the
Universities of Sydney, Queensland and Chicago,
and has had wide experience as a social work
practitioner, teacher and researcher. Faith is
President of the Northern Ireland Reminiscence
Network, and her extensive work and publications
inform the basis of all training delivered by the
Reminiscence Network Northern Ireland.

PAM SCHWEITZER

Pam Schweitzer is a writer, theatre director, trainer and lecturer. She is the founder of Age Exchange Theatre Trust and the European Reminiscence Network. She has created and directed 30 professional theatre productions based on recordings of older people's memories about social history of the 20th century. She opened the world's first Reminiscence Centre in London in 1987. She has published widely on her work, and written her own books and manuals on working creatively with older people. She now lives in Sydney, Australia.

ANNE BASTING

Anne Davis Basting (PhD) is an educator, scholar, artist and 2016 MacArthur Fellow. For over 15 years, she has developed and researched methods for embedding the arts into long-term care. She is author/producer of nearly a dozen plays and performances. She is founder and President of the award-winning non-profit TimeSlips Creative Storytelling and was Founding Director of UWM's Center on Age and Community from 2003 to 2013. She lives in Milwaukee with her husband and their two sons. She published *Forget Memory* in 2009.

STEPHEN POST

Stephen Garrard Post is a researcher, public speaker, professor, and best-selling author currently teaching at Stony Brook University School of Medicine (2008–). He is an elected member of several medical associations. His book *The Moral Challenge of Alzheimer Disease: Ethical Issues from Diagnosis to Dying* (Johns Hopkins University Press, 2nd edition 2000) was designated a 'medical classic of the century' by the British Medical Journal. He is a recipient of the US Alzheimer's Association 'distinguished service award'.

JULIAN HUGHES

Professor Julian Hughes is the first RICE Professor of Old Age Psychiatry, based at the Royal United Hospital, Bath. He is involved in academic research examining palliative care in dementia. He is a Fellow of both the Royal College of Psychiatrists and of the Royal College of Physicians of Edinburgh. He serves on several committees of the Royal College of Psychiatrists and advised NICE about guidelines on Dementia and on the Care of Dying Adults in the Last Days of Life. He is the author of numerous publications.

PETER WHITEHOUSE

Peter J. Whitehouse, MD, PhD and MA (Bioethics) is Professor of Neurology. He is the author (with Danny George) of *The Myth of Alzheimer's: What You Aren't Being Told About Today's Most Dreaded Diagnosis*. Currently he is an advisor in strategic innovation at Baycrest, a geriatric care complex and brain research institute in Toronto. He is clinically active at the Joseph Foley Elder Health Center caring for individuals with concerns about their cognitive abilities as they age and co-founder of the Intergenerational School.

This book is called *The Story of Dementia.* Are there other stories to be told, and if so, what should be included?

What aspects do you find hopeful in this story?

What aspects do you find
surprising?

Look at the collage of media
expressions. Would you describe
your experience of dementia in any
of those terms?

Will you read more about the
people mentioned in this book?
Who did you find most interesting?

What kind of person should be a
spokesperson for people with
dementia?

What role can a writer play in our public health and care system?

Do you use the words 'sufferer' and 'afflicted' when talking about people with dementia? Why does John disagree with these words?

Mary Marshall advocates using the term 'rehabilitation' to cover some aspects of dementia care. What advantages could this have?

Speaking as a person with dementia Christine Bryden says 'You can restore our personhood, and give us a sense of being needed and valued.' How is this to be achieved?

Can you name 3 to 5
characteristics that make
you different from others,
as Faith Gibson suggests?

'People flourish when they
feel respected and heard' –
Steve Sabat. How can we ensure
people feel respected and heard?
Think of a time when you felt
respected and heard.

'We are giving people false hope'.
What do you think of Peter
Whitehouse's characterisation of
the Alzheimer movement in
these words?

Who might you recommend this
book to?

Do you think the book is 'so biased
as to be a distortion of the truth'
or do you think it tells a true
Story of Dementia?

Some other books published by **LUATH** PRESS

**Dementia Positive:
A Handbook Based on
Lived Experiences:
For everyone wishing to
improve the lives of those
with dementia**
John Killick
ISBN 978-1-1910021-50-7
£9.99 PBK

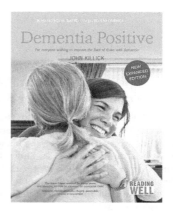

Dementia is a mysterious
condition. It frightens many of
us. When we are confronted
with someone with it we feel
helpless. This is not how it has
to be.

John Killick, in this thought-
provoking and warm-hearted
book, challenges these
assumptions. He shows us ways
in which we can help, and make
lives better for all concerned.
He writes out of two decades
of experience of working with
people with dementia and their
carers, friends and supporters.
He also shares with us the
views of many of the people he
has encountered on his journey.
Now containing a new section
that addresses the difficult
questions posed to the author
after the first edition, *Dementia
Positive* is an essential handbook
for anyone living with a
dementia diagnosis, as well as
dementia care professionals
and relatives seeking further
insight into the condition.

*A wonderful book that empowers,
demystifies and inspires.*
TANYA MYERS, *Carer*

*A must-read as a step towards
making life better for people with
dementia.*
DR SANDRA DAVIS, *Gerontologist*

*This book is exceptional... it says
exactly what I think and try to say.*
KEITH OLIVER, *Person with Dementia*

*The book I have wanted for many
years.*
SUE BENSON, *Editor of Journal of
Dementia Care*

*Intimate, conversational... hugely
accessible.*
JANICE H GALLOWAY

*Dementia Positive: A Handbook
Based on Lived Experiences* is part
of the national Reading Well
Books on Prescription scheme
for England delivered by The
Reading Agency and the Society
of Chief Librarians with funding
from Arts Council England.
www.reading-well.org.uk

Details of these and other books published by Luath Press
can be found at: **www.luath.co.uk**

Luath Press Limited
committed to publishing well written books worth reading

LUATH PRESS takes its name from Robert Burns, whose little collie Luath (*Gael.,* swift or nimble) tripped up Jean Armour at a wedding and gave him the chance to speak to the woman who was to be his wife and the abiding love of his life. Burns called one of 'The Twa Dogs' Luath after Cuchullin's hunting dog in Ossian's *Fingal.* Luath Press was established in 1981 in the heart of Burns country, and now resides a few steps up the road from Burns' first lodgings on Edinburgh's Royal Mile. Luath offers you distinctive writing with a hint of unexpected pleasures.

Most bookshops in the UK, the US, Canada, Australia, New Zealand and parts of Europe either carry our books in stock or can order them for you. To order direct from us, please send a £sterling cheque, postal order, international money order or your credit card details (number, address of cardholder and expiry date) to us at the address below. Please add post and packing as follows: UK – £1.00 per delivery address; overseas surface mail – £2.50 per delivery address; overseas airmail – £3.50 for the first book to each delivery address, plus £1.00 for each additional book by airmail to the same address. If your order is a gift, we will happily enclose your card or message at no extra charge.

Luath Press Limited
543/2 Castlehill
The Royal Mile
Edinburgh EH1 2ND
Scotland

Telephone: 0131 225 4326 (24 hours)
email: sales@luath.co.uk
Website: www.luath.co.uk